Seasons
of the
Desert

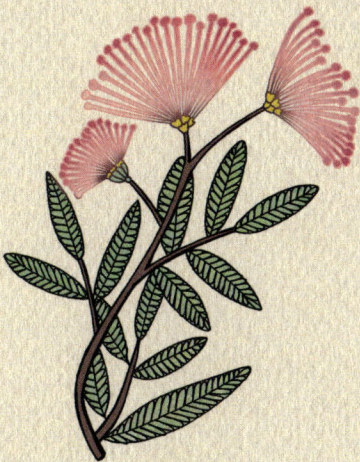

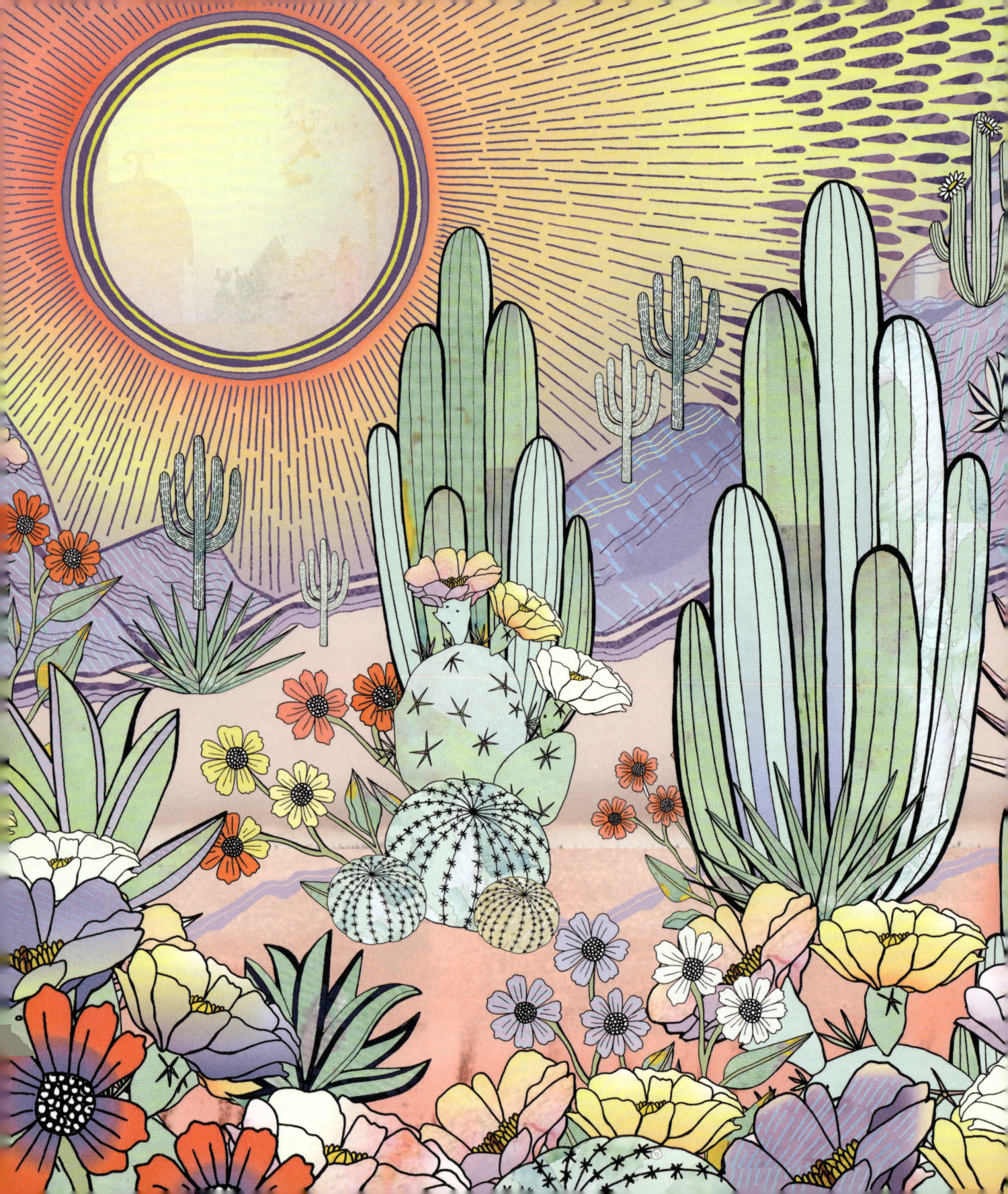

Seasons of the Desert

The Wellness Wisdom of Southwestern Native Plants

Sonoran Rosie

wellfleet
press

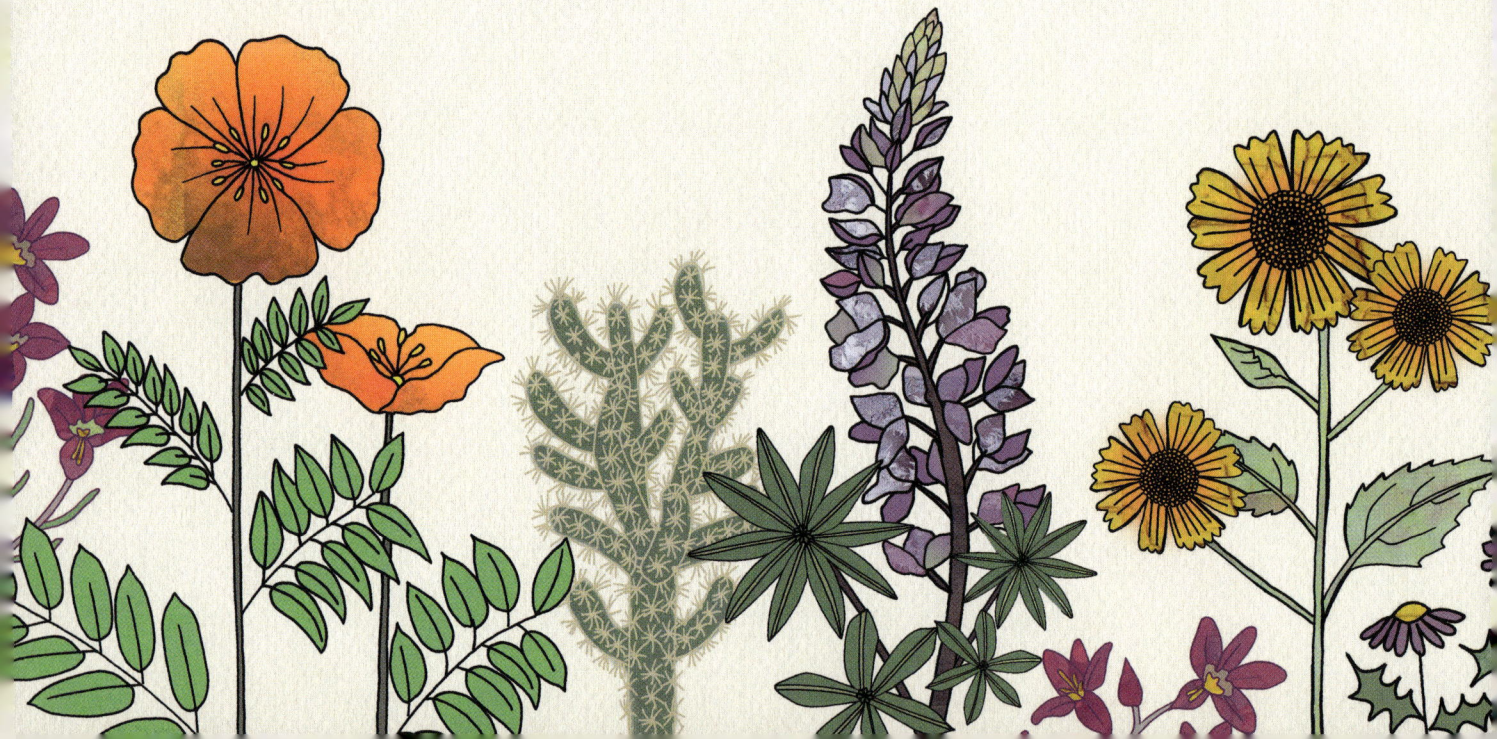

Contents

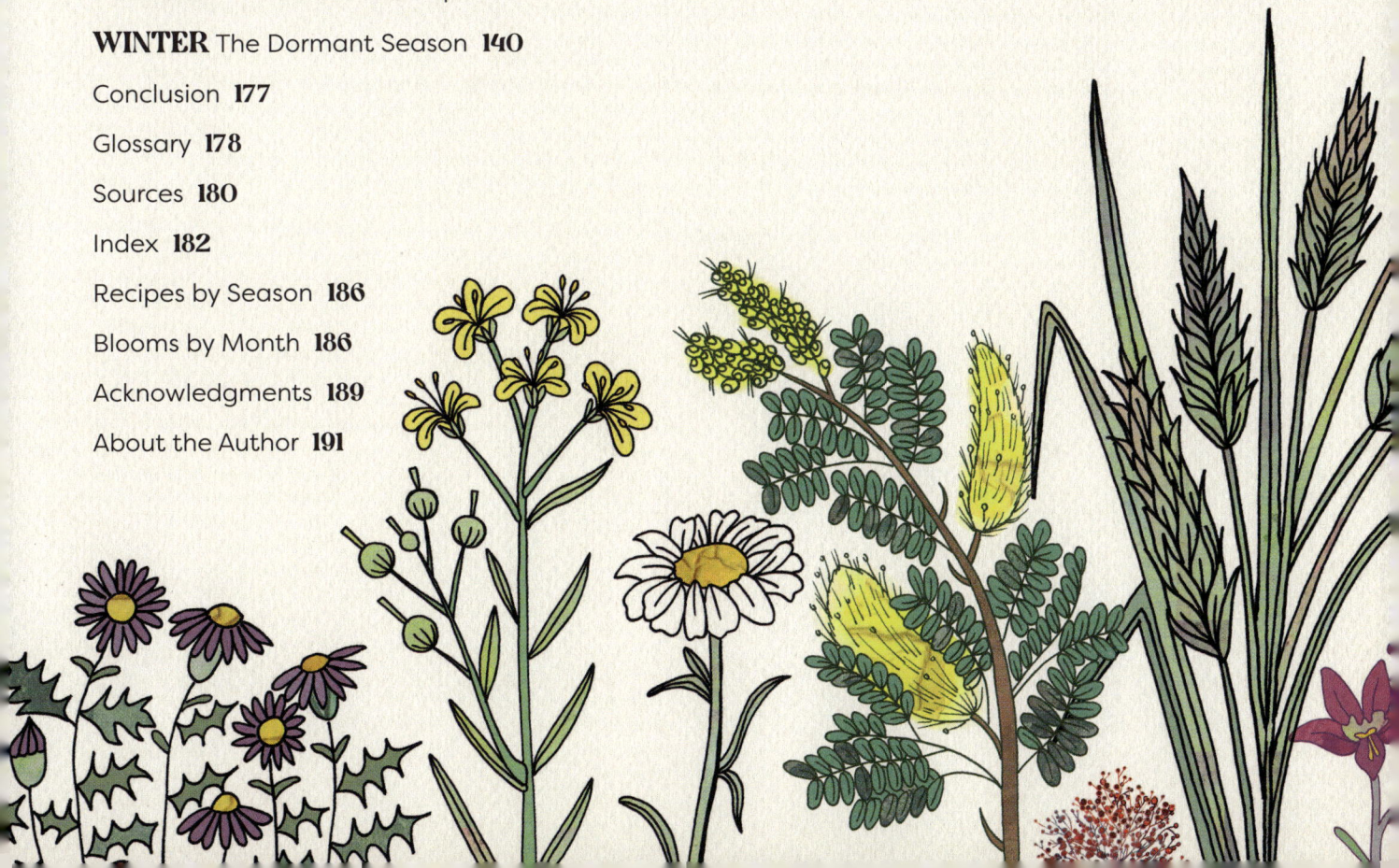

Preface

I was born and raised in Arizona. After visiting Tucson in 2007, I decided to move from Phoenix to make Tucson my forever home. Tucson is where I found community, nature, and inspiration. Starting with an interest in gardening and houseplants in my twenties and an endless curiosity for learning, I began to listen to the signs from the universe and started learning more about the desert plants that surrounded me. I was always hiking and enjoying the outdoors. I slowly started to see that so many of the plants in the Sonoran Desert were edible and began learning how to identify and forage these desert foods. This began an intense, lifelong passion for all that is the desert.

I began searching for local natural perfumes or skincare that included desert plants, but was only able to find creosote bush salves. My problem-solving skills spurred me to begin experimenting with creosote bush and desert wildflowers, with an aim to bring the magical scents of the desert closer to me. I knew I needed more guidance and was introduced to a local herbalist in Tucson with over twenty years of experience, Becki Garza of La Yerberia. I enjoyed working as an assistant to Becki, helping her make her herbal creations and learning along the way.

After a year of assisting, I felt I had the information I needed to create everyday skincare, haircare, natural perfumes, and other self-care products out of desert plants. There wasn't an all-natural line like this on the market, and I was inspired to take on this task to create it myself. I shared those early products with friends, and quickly more and more people began asking to purchase them. The universe aligned to assist and with the support of my partner at the time, I was able to invest in kicking off my business, Sonoran Rosie, out of my home.

After growing up in poverty, struggling, and feeling isolated most of my life, I wanted to connect with my local creative community, and Sonoran Rosie was a great way to start participating in local makers markets. I made so many close friends, and this drove my passion for cultivating community. I believe that the biggest issue facing society today is our lack of community and connectedness. After three years of successfully running my business, I collaborated with a few local makers to create a local pop-up market called Desert Air Market. This is a biannual market for local makers to showcase and sell their creations while uplifting local nonprofits and taking part in creative community mixers. My aim was to create something that wasn't purely based on revenue and had a positive impact on the community as a whole.

As I grew closer with my local creative community, by 2022, I had outgrown my home workspace (with one employee) and began searching for a space where I could both work on and sell my creations. I found a lovely, large space in downtown Tucson and started creating a vision for a shop that was like no other in the city: an inviting space with lots of color, local art, vintage clothing, and plants, with room for artistic workshops, all with a Sonoran Desert twist.

Arizona Poppy was born in May 2022, named after a desert wildflower that only blooms after plentiful monsoon rain, which speaks to the importance of rarities and abundance in the desert. Arizona Poppy has become a pivotal part of the Tucson small business community, hosting workshops and events, donating to important local organizations, and continually supporting the local creative community. I now have a team of people who work together to continue to grow both the Sonoran Rosie line and Arizona Poppy.

I currently live alone with my two dogs and my garden and spend most of my time exploring and foraging in the desert. I connected with my biological father, who lives in southern Utah, in December 2023 and have been growing a new relationship with him and his side of the family ever since. That has also given me a beautiful opportunity to start exploring the Mojave Desert. I have amazing friends and relationships, and I cherish my community. I continue to have daily gratitude for all that the desert has provided me. Plants and nature have played such a large role in healing my past traumas, and though I know I have overcome a lot, I am always growing, just like the plants I know and love.

I am not a studied botanist, and so I have written this book from my lived experiences with these plants. I hope to bring awareness to desert plants in a relatable way, so terminology sometimes used in this book can be more descriptive than scientifically accurate.

The indexes at the back of the book can help you quickly refer to recipes and specific plants you may be interested in, and include an at-a-glance guide to the flowers that typically bloom each month. This calendar does not account for plants that do not have a concrete blooming season, so keep the full profiles handy for identification in the field.

I truly believe in the power of nature and that we can learn so much about ourselves through slowing down, appreciating the small things, and getting outside!

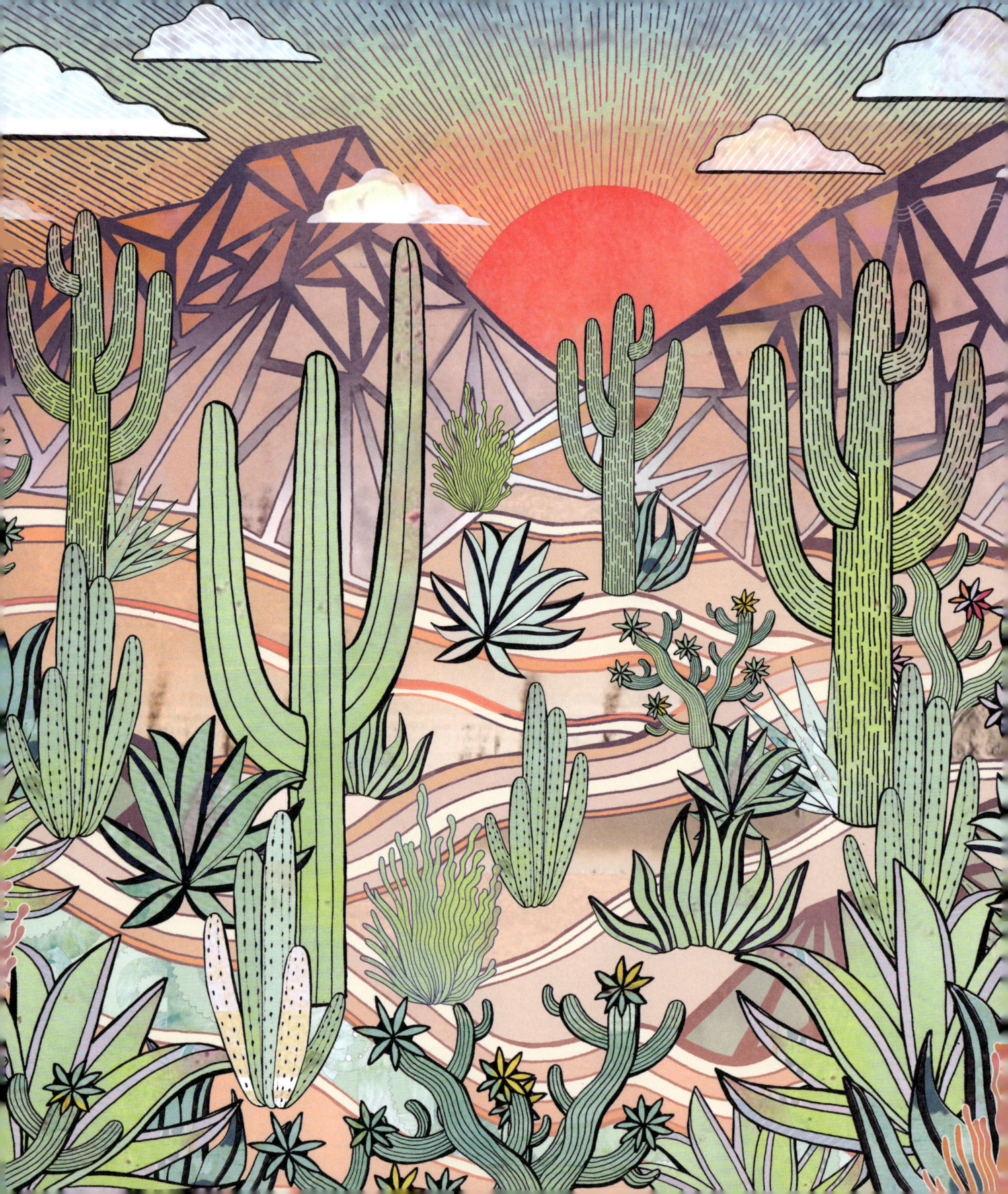

The Sonoran Desert

When we imagine a desert, we think of a desolate, dry place with vast mountains. While, yes, there are some areas like this, the Sonoran Desert encompasses so much more. It is a unique, lush, awe-inspiring place. It is filled with rare plants that can only be found here and seasons that vary dramatically. The main scientific distinction of the Sonoran Desert compared to other deserts is the presence of leguminous trees and columnar cacti like saguaro, which can only be found in a small area in the Sonoran Desert in central and southern Arizona.

The Sonoran Desert has many different ecosystems in one geographical location. It expands west through the lower portion of California, east through Arizona to parts of New Mexico, north almost to Utah, and south through Sonora and Baja California, Mexico. This desert includes all of the world's biomes in one region! My experience and the focus of this book are in the heart of the Sonoran Desert, but let's talk about some of the main biomes that surround and make up the biodiversity of this enchanting land. However, keep in mind that these biomes can blend into each other or even contain little pockets of different biomes.

Temperate Deciduous Forest and Sky Islands

These higher-elevation areas scattered throughout the Sonoran Desert contain a mixture of riparian trees, evergreens, and oaks. We call them the sky islands of the Sonoran Desert because they are high mountain peaks that contain a completely different biome than the surrounding desert or thornscrub foothills. There are four full seasons in temperate deciduous forests marked by regrowth in the spring, warm temperatures and lots of rain in the summer, fallen leaves in autumn, and snow in the winter. Sky islands are beautiful retreats from the hotter, drier climates below. Here in Tucson, we have two nearby sky islands: Mt. Lemmon and Madera Canyon/Mt. Wrightson. It is truly magical to take a drive up one of these mountains and see the biomes change before your eyes.

Grassland

The desert-grassland biome is a transitional landscape that is a cross between prairies and deserts. It is especially lush during and after the monsoon season. It contains many native grasses, succulents, and shrubs. We can find desert grassland between desert biomes and chaparral biomes scattered throughout the Sonoran Desert and in the slopes and valleys below mountains.

Chaparral

The desert-chaparral biome is characterized by dry, hot summers and wet winters. The plants and wildlife that live here are well adapted to going without water for long periods. The exact definition of chaparral is "vegetation consisting chiefly of tangled shrubs and thorny bushes," which is true for our desert-chaparral biome. Scrubby bushes with waxy leaves to retain moisture and short, thorny trees like mesquite make up the majority of the landscape. Desert-chaparral biomes are found along the lower slopes of the sky islands and in Baja California. Wildfire is a regular occurrence and is necessary for the soil and some seeds to germinate.

Desert

The common denominator of all deserts is a severe lack of water. Water here is only available for short times after sporadic rainfall, mostly in the summer during the monsoon season. The landscape is sparse and filled with tough, resilient plants like cacti that absorb as much water as they can during a rainstorm to store for future dry spells. All plant life in the desert biome has some way to retain water. Wildlife is also well adapted to long drought periods. The temperature fluctuates dramatically in the desert, even within a single day. There can be a 30°F (-1°C) difference between day and night. A great example of the desert biome is the area in and surrounding Phoenix, Arizona.

Thornscrub

This biome mainly consists of small, thorny trees such as velvet mesquite, vines, and cacti, all intertangling to create dense vegetation. This is an intermediate biome between tropical forest and desert. The temperatures here are rarely freezing and consist of wet and dry seasons. The Tucson area has many thornscrub biomes throughout it.

Riparian Communities

These areas are not considered biomes but instead isolated areas where perennial water is near the surface. Riparian communities exist in zones along the banks of rivers, marshes, and lakes—anywhere water collects—and are characterized by water plants like cattails and watercress, fish like Arizona minnows, and tons of wildlife not normally seen in the drier areas of the Sonoran Desert. Riparian communities are truly lush oases. The Santa Cruz River in and near Tucson used to flow year-round, but after many years of groundwater usage, it dried up, only flowing when it rains. Efforts to restore the river using water reclamation have created a riparian community along its banks.

A Note on Tucson

Since most of my interactions with the Sonoran Desert revolve around Tucson, I would be remiss if I did not include a little history of this area, the heart of the Sonoran Desert. The free-flowing Santa Cruz River was what drew Indigenous peoples to the area thousands of years ago. The Hohokam people (ancestors of the Tohono O'odham) created settlements along many different riverbanks in the Sonoran Desert and lived in flourishing communities. They created beautiful pottery and were known for their advanced irrigation systems. The Tohono O'odham carried on these traditions, looking to the stars to know when to plant and harvest crops, and for important rites and ceremonies. They grew (and continue to grow) tepary beans, squash, corn, and melons, and wild-harvested plants like saguaro fruit, mesquite beans, and cholla buds. Colonizers would not know about the edible and medicinal plants here in the desert without the knowledge of the Tohono O'odham.

A major settlement of the Tohono O'odham was located at the base of Chuk Son, or black mountain, known today as "A" Mountain in central Tucson. This mountain served as a lookout point from which to oversee crops along the floodplains of the Santa Cruz, and spot incoming danger. The Spanish were the first colonizers to come into contact with the Tohono O'odham and Pima Indigenous peoples in 1687. Over time, through wars and treaties, the land was eventually taken over by the United States, leaving a small reservation for the Tohono O'odham. The base of "A" Mountain became a landfill. This disrespect for the land and its first peoples is something that we continually see throughout the history of not just the United States but colonizing nations in general. It is heartbreaking what we have done to this desert that was once such a lush paradise and how we decimated and removed the people who knew how to love and work with nature. But I believe we can become caretakers once again.

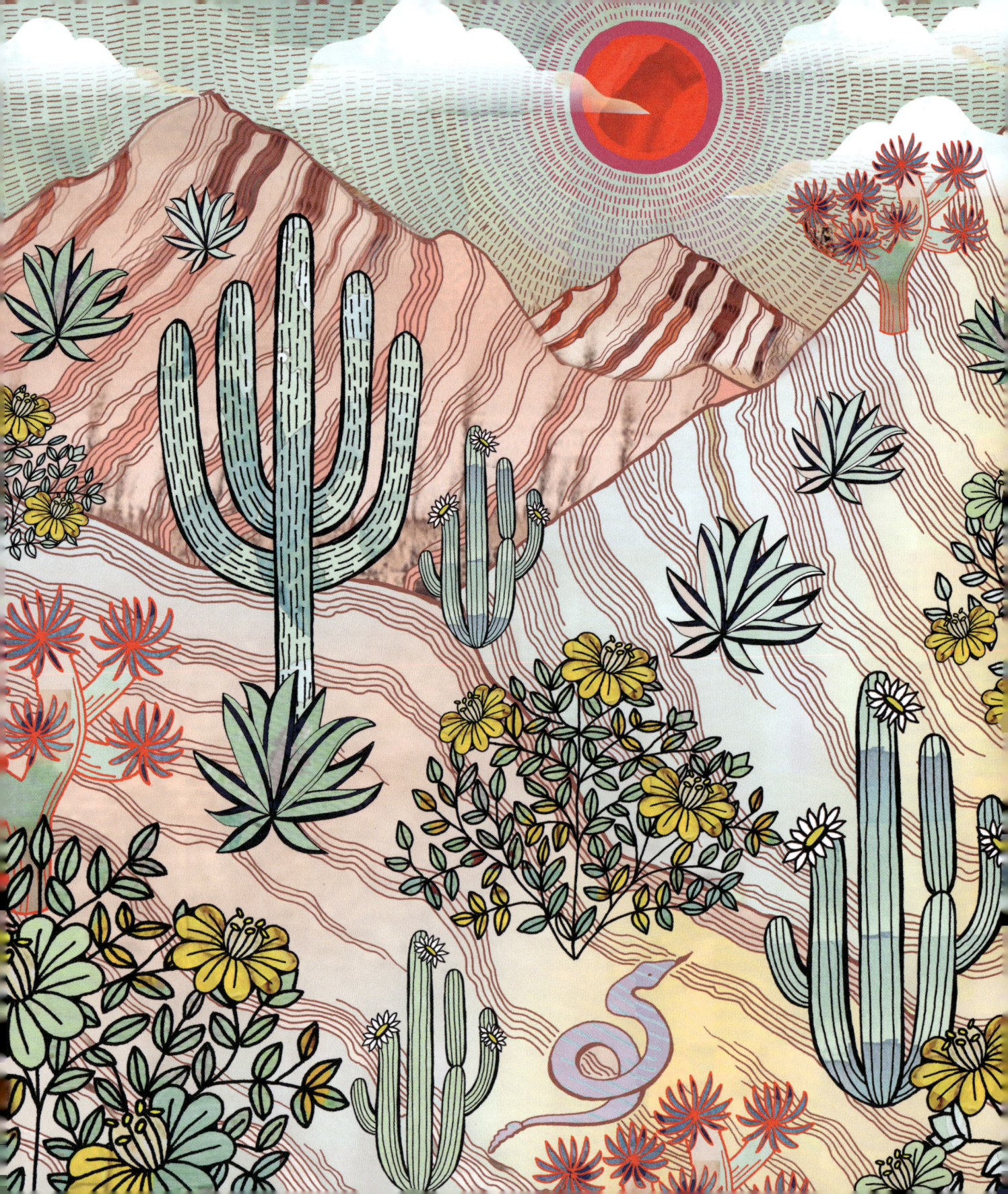

Sustainable Foraging

We think of the desert as barren, but there is an abundance of food and life in the Sonoran Desert, especially in southern Arizona. This unique landscape is awe-inspiring but can also be harsh. To that end, there is much to consider when adventuring into the desert and foraging.

The desert contains many different cacti with varying levels of spines and glochids (small, hairlike thorns that are highly irritating to the skin), holes that are home to many different creatures, venomous creatures during some parts of the year, little to no water in some areas, and extreme weather conditions. This is why we must start with protection. The essentials for desert life during any season include sunscreen, a large hat, plenty of water, breathable long sleeves and pants, hiking boots, a back-up phone charger or battery, and a first aid kit that must include tweezers and a tourniquet. The first few are pretty self-explanatory, but tweezers are for any number of cacti that you could accidentally come in contact with, and a tourniquet is for possible rattlesnake bites, to avoid the venom spreading quickly while you seek medical attention. (Rattlesnakes are out and about from the late spring until the end of summer—they are hibernating the rest of the year.)

I personally have never been bitten by a rattlesnake, even though I encounter them often every summer, because I am always looking down—which brings us to the next point. *Always* look down. The wildlife here in the desert just wants to be left alone. It is our responsibility to be aware of our surroundings, always watching and listening to ensure we aren't disturbing them or encroaching on their homes and territories. Snakes may seem scary but are actually pretty docile and just want to go on their way. When I come across any snake, I just walk a big half circle around it, or I go the other way. Rattlesnakes can be hard to spot, so it's good not to have earbuds or headphones in, so you can also hear the telltale rattle or listen for movement among the brush.

Every tool you use will be different depending on what you are foraging, but if you live the life of a forager, it's good to keep the essentials in your vehicle or backpack so you always have what you need. These include a woven basket, tongs, paper bags, clippers, a foldable bag, and gloves.

Just like the tools, scouting locations for your foraging also depends on the season and what you are looking for. Some basic guidelines to follow:

1. Stay away from areas that are right next to roads. Heavy metals from vehicles' exhaust can settle on the plants and cause health issues for the plant—and yourself!

2. Find areas where the plants look healthy and green (usually near water sources). Foraging from a struggling plant is never a good idea because you could harm the plant further. A healthy plant usually has more to offer, including calmer energy and a more positive experience overall.

3. Stay away from national parks and private property. Most national parks prohibit foraging because there are many people out there that will be disrespectful or take too much.

Showing respect and gratitude to the plants you are foraging is of utmost importance. The Sonoran Desert can be far more than arid, with so much abundance to offer us and the wildlife. Slowing down and taking your time to connect with the plants and their energy will bring you into communion with the plants. I always observe and admire them before I forage. Being in nature really helps ground me, and I give credit for so much of the healing I have done over the years to the plants and the greater connection between us all. I never rush through foraging (even when needed for creating products for my business) because the foraging experience is not just taking, but appreciating. Thanking each plant after we forage what we need from it lets the universe know we are grateful.

So, how much do we forage from a plant? Again, every plant will be different and it depends on what we are looking to forage. My rule of thumb is never more than 10 percent of a single plant or fruit. If foraging the entire plant is called for, then I forage just one plant per every twenty that remains, to protect the area from overharvesting. Why is overharvesting harmful? We as humans tend to spend a lot of time consuming thoughtlessly and this is not how nature intended us to live. When we over-consume, we not only damage the plant and the ecosystem, but we leave little to nothing for the wildlife that depends on these food sources, fewer chances for the plant to seed and propagate, and less for ourselves and the environment as a whole in the future. Thinking big picture is essential to foraging.

If you are foraging a plant regularly, you should wait at least six months before revisiting a plant, but a year is ideal. I regularly forage creosote bush (chaparral) branches (of about 12 inches, or 30 cm, long) for our Creosote Shower Bundles, which help bring the scent of desert rain into people's homes. I call what I am doing pruning because I trim off the tallest branches, only a few from each bush, and then I don't return for at least six months. Because I have been following these methods for years, I have returned to bushes I have foraged from and found they are always bushier, healthier, and happier than some of the surrounding plants that I haven't foraged from. I have developed a close relationship with certain bushes and love to see that what they are giving to me also helps them thrive.

Wild desert foraging can be tough but so rewarding, as long as we are mindful in all we do and understand all the ways we benefit from wild plants. That way, we can develop a mutual loving relationship between us and the land we live on.

Spring

The Desert in Bloom

March through May

After a short winter with plenty of rainfall, desert dwellers (especially us plant lovers) eagerly keep watch for the coming spring; nature giving us the telltale sign of little sprouts blanketing the desert floor. We see glimpses of titillating color toward the end of February; however, the desert shows its full glory in March. Rolling hills of bright-orange poppies with their translucent petals flittering in the wind; the resinous creosote bushes sprinkled with tiny yellow flowers; globemallows lining the roadways like little soldiers, standing tall, keeping watch over the desert; woolly wildflowers like the wild heliotropes and the fiddleheads finding protection on slopes and near desert shrubs and trees; electric-yellow dancing desert marigolds and brittlebush mimicking the sunlight: intense, bursting, and bright.

Spring is an exciting time. It is the first of the natural seasons and people come to the Sonoran Desert in droves during springtime to witness the magic of the desert in bloom. There are so many wildflowers to see during spring that I never seem to go everywhere I had planned to. There are many areas in and around Tucson and Phoenix that are wildflower destinations, such as Picacho Peak State Park, Lost Dutchman's State Park, Catalina State Park, and South Mountain Park, to name a few. Even while driving along the highways, you will see brilliant displays of brittlebush lining the ditches. Once every few years, with enough winter rain, we have a superbloom (an extraordinary display of fields of wildflowers like California poppies, Arizona lupine, globemallow, and brittlebush).

The desert is truly a magical place in the spring—and is, by far, my favorite of the seasons—and it never lasts long enough. The Pascua Yaqui tribe describes a flower world that is a land of paradise, parallel to our own, a kind of spiritual metaphor that could have been inspired by the powerful magic of spring here in the Sonoran Desert. I am always overtaken by the beauty of desert wildflowers; their soft, demure presence among a harsh landscape has always inspired me. I am always a little depressed when I see the spring wildflowers start to dry up, but I like to believe that spring can live with us always as a constant glimmer of hope.

This season will be full of wildflower identification. There is just something about admiring flowers that creates feelings of calm and peace within us.

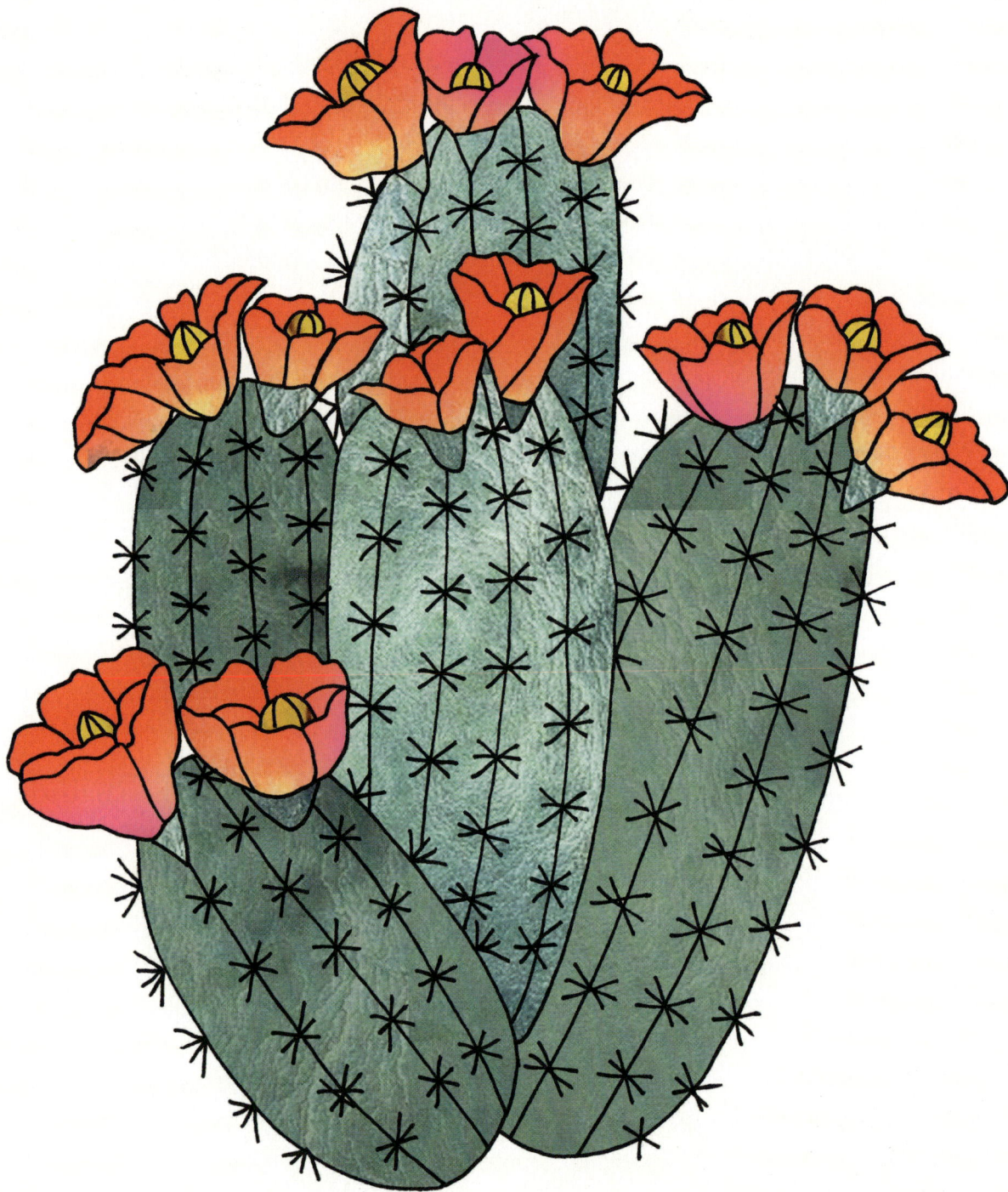

Arizona Hedgehog Cactus

Echinocereus arizonicus

Appearance: This rare and gorgeous, small, dark-green columnar cactus grows low to the ground, up to about 16 inches (41 cm) tall and 10 inches (25 cm) in diameter in clustered stems ranging from four to twenty stems. Its spines are smooth and short. Flowers erupt along the sides of the stem and are a striking crimson color. The stout flowers measure 2 inches (5 cm) in diameter and 3 inches (7.5 cm) in length. The color of this flower against the rocky, brown desert floor is remarkable.

Habitat: Found in a small range in the Madrean woodlands and Interior Chaparral communities in Gila and Pinal counties in central Arizona. Grows in stable bedrock or rock fields. I have personally seen them growing wild along the rocky mountainsides of the Superstition Mountains just outside of Phoenix.

Blooming season: Late April to mid-May.

Lifespan: This cactus has been observed to live nine years but could possibly live longer.

Threats: This cactus is on the endangered list and protected under Arizona law. There have been efforts made by the Center for Plant Conservation and Desert Botanical Garden to repopulate areas that were previously decimated by road construction, mining, and wildfires with this cactus.

Environmental role: The Arizona hedgehog cactus helps prevent soil erosion with its root grip. It also provides shelter and food for many animals, such as bats, bees, and various birds.

Foraging: All hedgehog cactus fruit is edible, but because it's an endangered plant, I would discourage anyone from eating this specific variety unless you plan to propagate the seeds. Indigenous cultures used this cactus to heal wounds.

Plant friends: Engelmann's hedgehog cactus, Arizona rainbow cactus.

Arizona Lupine

Lupinus arizonicus

Appearance: These easily recognizable beauties have long flower spikes with small palmate compound leaves at the bottom of the stalk. The flowers are pea shaped and can range from twenty to fifty flowers per spike. The flower colors of each plant vary widely, from whitish to magenta to a bluish purple.

Habitat: Found in the Sonoran and Mojave Deserts at lower elevations (under 3,600 feet or 1,097 m) in rocky desert hillsides or sandy soils, and often seen near creosote bush communities. Arizona lupine is often seen growing in droves off the sides of roadways.

Blooming season: January to May.

Lifespan: Annual wildflower (completes its lifespan in one year, from germination to bloom to seed to decay).

Environmental role: These gorgeous wildflowers are attractive to pollinators such as butterflies, moths, and native bees. Their seeds are consumed by small rodents and birds. They are a main attraction in a lot of popular spring desert wildflower destination locations. These wildflowers also replenish nutrients in the soil, making them great for restoring native ecosystems.

Foraging: Oils that promote skin health can be extracted from lupine seeds. This flower is not recommended for herbal uses as it has a toxic chemical that must be removed from the seed before consuming. I personally love to forage lupine flowers for making wildflower bouquets, both fresh and dried, as this flower is abundant in the springtime.

Plant friends: Coulter's lupine, Bajada lupine, Hill's lupine.

Desert Dispatch

Arizona lupines are great additions to desert-wildflower bouquets when kept in water. When foraging, find stems that have plenty of open blooms on them and trim at the base, making sure not to damage the bottom portion of the plant so it can continue to produce flowers.

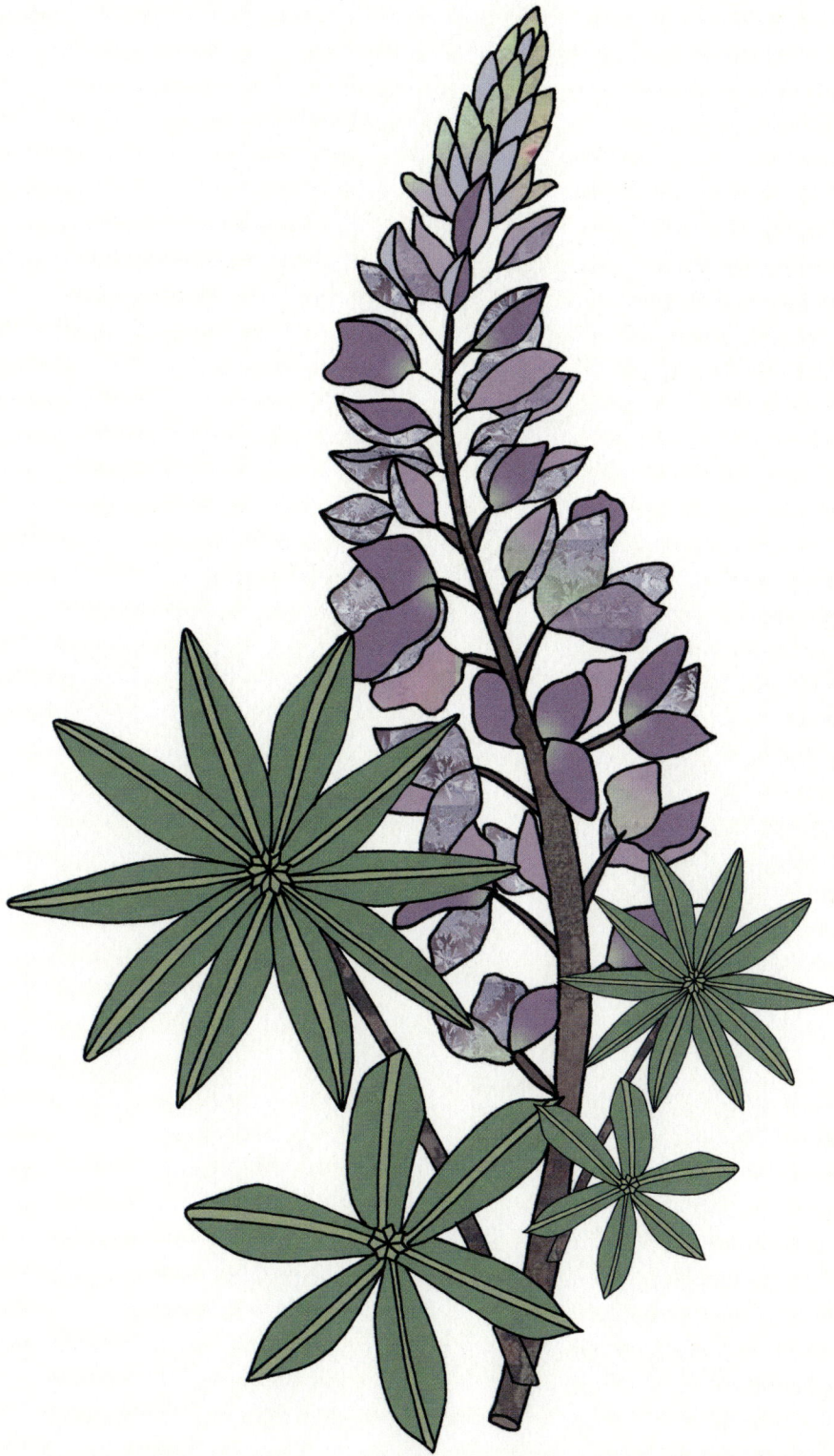

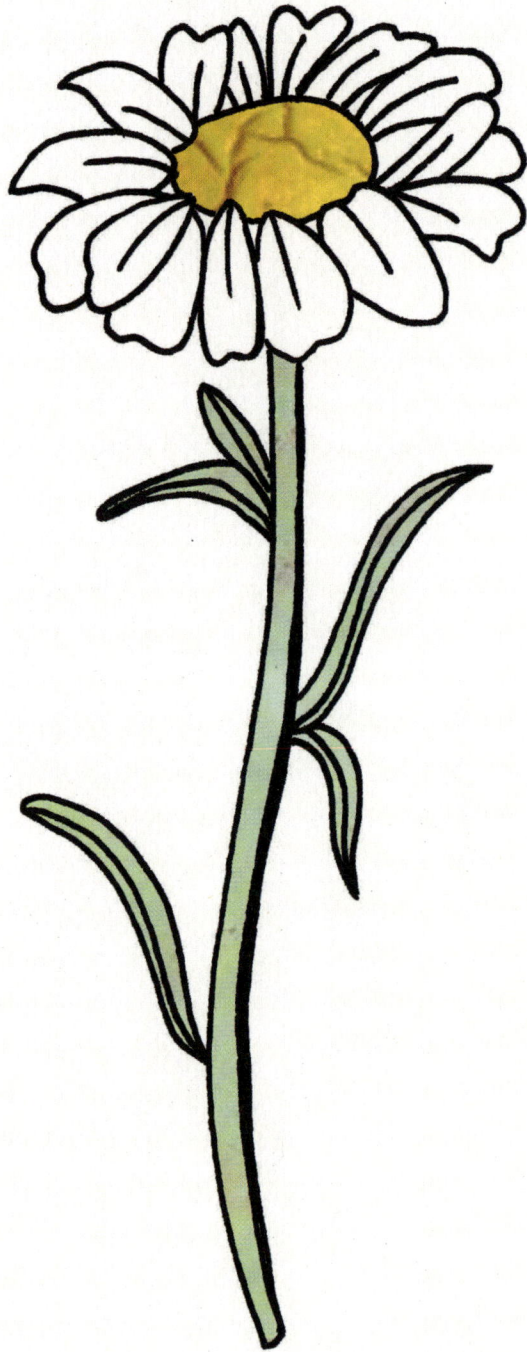

Blackfoot Daisy

Melampodium leucanthum

Appearance: The showy flowers on this wildflower bush have small white petals that bloom on the tip of a slender stem. They have thin, lancelike green leaves that are covered in fine hairs. They grow low to the ground in clumps about 1 to 2 feet (30.5 to 61 cm) across and rarely over 6 inches (15 cm) high.

Habitat: They grow all over the Southwest of the United States and can be found in a range of soil types, from rocky to caliche.

Blooming season: March to November. I love these flowers because they bloom so often throughout the year.

Lifespan: These flowers are perennial, meaning they can grow for an infinite amount of time depending on water sources, but in a wild environment they tend to dry up in the summer and come back with regular rain.

Environmental role: These native wildflowers are great for pollinators and require minimal water. They flower frequently and have a light honey scent. They are nontoxic to animals and are deer and rabbit resistant. Blackfoot daisies are the perfect ground coverage; ground-covering plants can help the entire area feel cooler, temperature-wise.

Foraging: This plant is thought to have anti-carcinogen properties but is not well known for its possible other herbal uses. This flower is nontoxic, so I use it to decorate things like bath bombs or soap. They are also perfect for pressing and drying, as they maintain their shape and color.

Plant friends: Blackfoot daisy is in the Asteraceae family, so it has so many relatives! Some here in Arizona are the common sunflower, desert zinnia, and desert marigold.

Brittlebush

Encelia farinosa

Appearance: This bushy, abundant desert wildflower puts on a real show in springtime. Growing in short bushes about 2 to 5 feet (0.6 to 1.5 m) tall, they have brittle, woody stems with light silvery-green leaves. Their flowers look very similar to small sunflowers or daisies, as they are bright yellow, a little larger than daisies, and grow in clusters. The flowers take over the top of the entire bush, making for a radiant display of yellow sprinkled throughout the desert.

Habitat: Brittlebush grows throughout southern Arizona, Southern California, southern Nevada, and throughout Sonora and Baja Mexico.

Blooming season: February through May.

Lifespan: One bush can live up to twenty years and easily clones itself through the root crown as well as plentiful seeds.

Environmental role: These bountiful bushes help prevent soil erosion and offer important nectar for pollinators and food through its seeds for wildlife. They have been used by Indigenous peoples to treat toothaches and chest pain. Their sap can be used as a natural glue.

Foraging: Brittlebush is abundant in the desert and is a plant I forage often because it is available almost year-round. I forage it for its amazing frankincense-like, musky scent and its beneficial, skin-healing properties. I use it in a natural perfume and in body cream. It also makes a great addition to spring wildflower bouquets.

Plant friends: Many other desert shrubs are in the same family and found in similar areas.

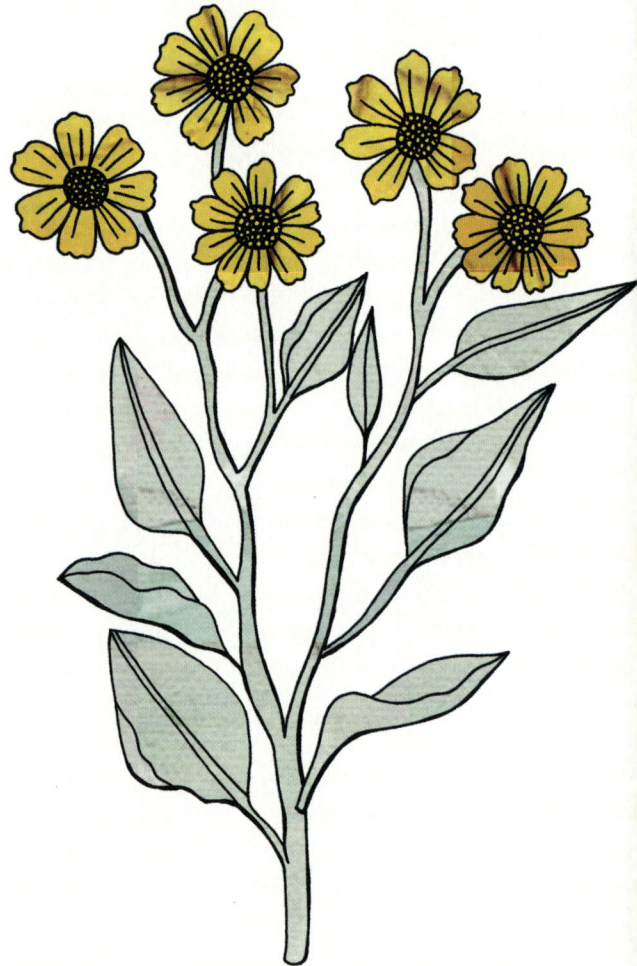

Brittlebush Hydrosol

You can create your very own healing face spray or natural scent by making a hydrosol out of foraged brittlebush leaves and small stems. Brittlebush is naturally hydrating and also has an amazing woody, almost smoky, scent. (Note: Only attempt this recipe if you have knowledge of or experience in using a distiller.)

MATERIALS

- Stovetop distiller (or alcohol still) intended for use with plant material
- Enough brittlebush leaves and small stems, cut up into ½-inch (1 cm) pieces, to fill the distiller pot
- Water, for the distiller (refer to the equipment's instructions)
- Glass or other nonplastic container, for the distilling process (refer to the equipment's instructions)
- 1-gallon (3.8 L) glass container, for storage
- Glass atomizer bottle, for spritzing
- Essential oil(s) (optional)

INSTRUCTIONS

1. Fill the distiller pot with brittlebush, following the equipment's instructions.

2. Each distiller is slightly different, so consult the distiller's instruction guide to set up your distiller in a way to extract the hydrosol from the plant material.

3. Bring up the temperature in the tank to over 200°F (93°C) to start the extraction process.

4. How long you run the distiller will depend on the size of your distiller and how much plant material you put in the pot. Because my distiller is small, I usually check and smell the hydrosol after 4 hours to see how strong the scent is, then I run it for another 4 hours, until the scent starts to get a little weaker, then I stop.

5. Store the hydrosol in the 1-gallon (3.8 L) glass container and let it sit for a couple of weeks, as the essential oils in the hydrosol will settle and become stronger.

6. Transfer the hydrosol to the glass atomizer bottle. You can add complementary essential oils, but it's also great on its own.

7. Spray it on your clothes, skin, face, and/or body.

California Poppies

Eschscholzia californica

Appearance: California poppies are easily the most recognizable desert wildflower. People visit the Sonoran Desert during the peak blooming season just to witness their beauty. They are known for blooming delicate bright-orange petals and blanketing large areas of the desert floor. They open their four-petal flowers when the sun is strongest, usually between 10 a.m. and 3 p.m., and are closed the rest of the day and on cloudy, windy days. They are usually about 8 inches (20 cm) tall, and the flower heads are no bigger than a clementine. They have bluish-green, feathery, fernlike leaves that grow very close together.

Habitat: Southwestern United States and northern Mexico; found in elevations up to 8,000 feet (2,438 m)

Blooming season: Late February through April.

Lifespan: Short-lived annual (only a few months every year).

Environmental role: California poppies are important for the environment in several ways. They are vital to pollinators as food sources and for habitat. They can convert nitrogen from the atmosphere into a form that plants can use, which enriches the soil. They also spread their seeds easily and the seeds can remain dormant in the ground until the right conditions arise for them to bloom.

Foraging: California poppy is an herbal medicine staple. It can reduce anxiety and promote relaxation and restful sleep. Its flower petals and stems can be used to create herbal tinctures and oxymels (a type of herbal extract using honey and vinegar). The petals are edible and are commonly used on salads and as decoration for baked goods. Please note that it is illegal to pick any plant on state or federal lands, but California poppies are easy to grow and you can get permission from land owners to forage. However you collect them, please forage in small amounts, as the environment needs these flowers more than we do.

Plant friends: Mexican gold poppy; not related to the opium poppy.

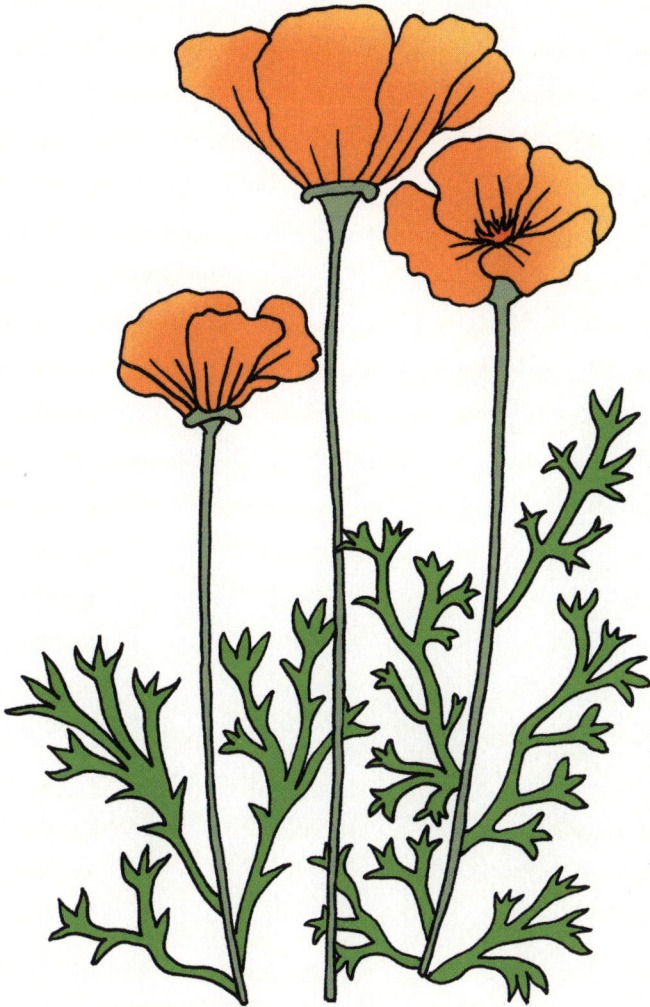

California Poppies

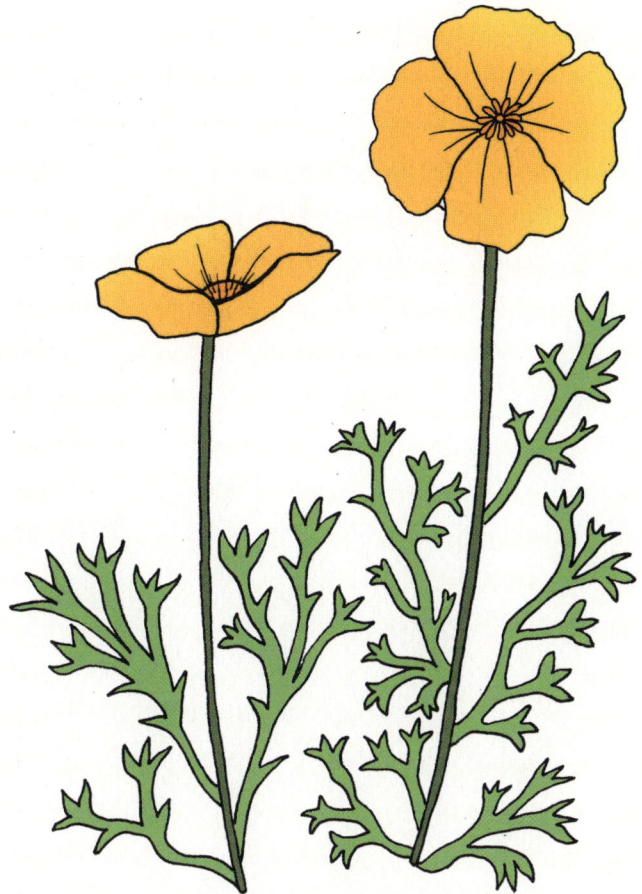

Mexican Gold Poppies

Difference Between California Poppies and Mexican Gold Poppies

- They are similar in range and properties. Mexican gold poppies are a subspecies of the California poppy.

- Mexican gold poppies are smaller and more yellow, while California poppies can be a variety of colors, including red, orange, and white.

- The undersides of California poppies have a small leaflike ring where the stem meets the petal (see illustration).

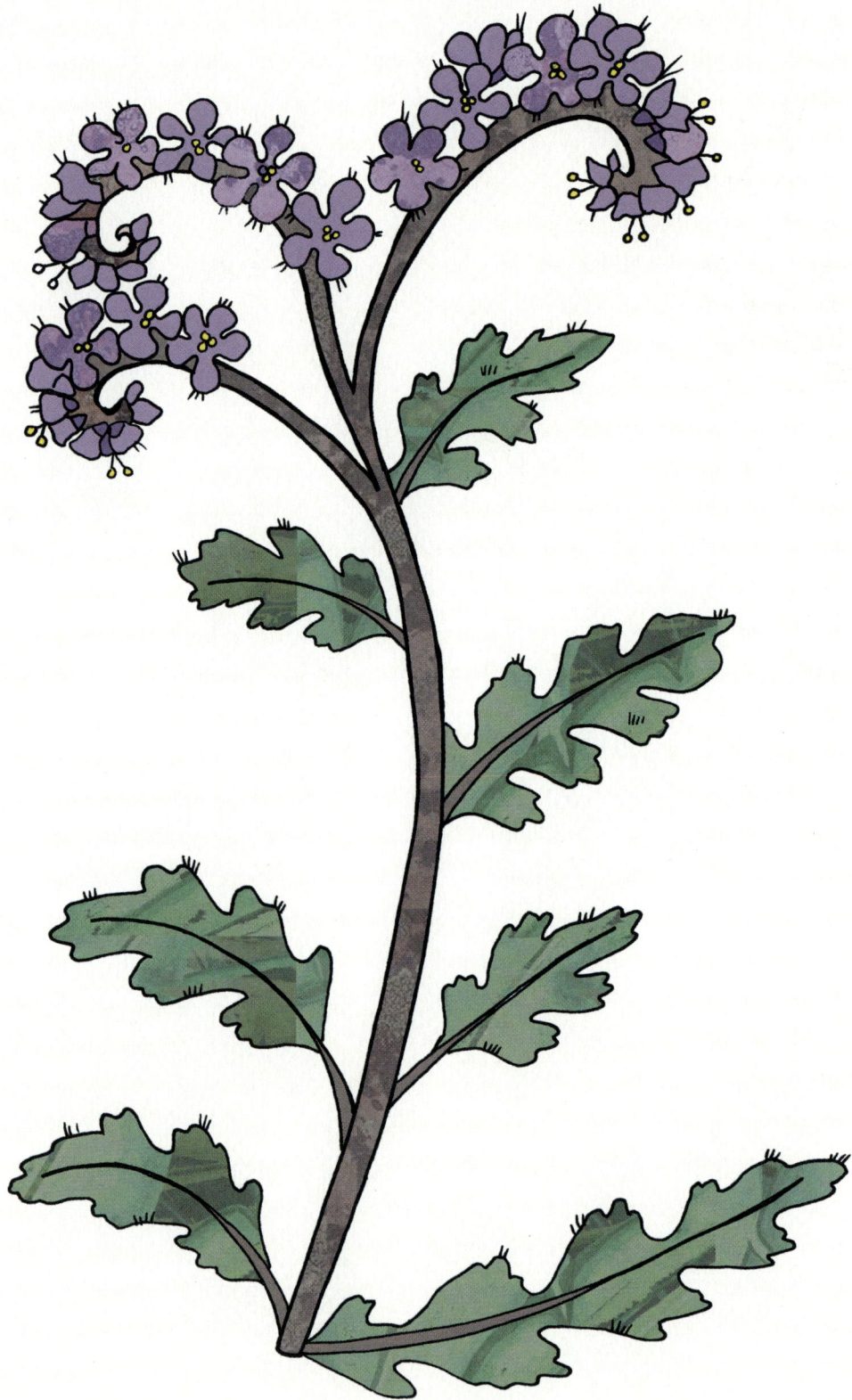

Cleftleaf Wild Heliotrope

Phacelia crenulata

Appearance: This prevalent desert wildflower grows erect stems covered with short hairs (to help protect it from wildlife and to retain moisture). The tip of its stems bud and form a curled tip from which the pretty little purple flowers bloom. They usually do not grow taller than 1.5 feet (46 cm), and have an onion-like odor. Their seeds disperse well and tend to grow many plants near each other, making for a beautiful display along the desert floor.

Habitat: Below 4,000 feet (1,219 m) elevation in the Sonoran, Chihuahuan, and Mojave Deserts, in plains, mesas, and foothills.

Blooming season: February through June.

Lifespan: Annual.

Environmental roles: Very important in the spring for native bees and vital for the native ecosystem.

Foraging: Wild heliotropes can be used to heal injuries in animals and can be used to soothe sore throats in humans. Their hairs can cause irritation if touched bare-handed and not properly prepared. I tend to leave these wildflowers be, as they have definitely caused me some uncomfortable itchiness in the past.

Plant friends: Any plant in the Phacelia genus, such as desert bluebells and Fremont's phacelia.

Desert Lavender

Hyptis emoryi

Appearance: This multistemmed, fragrant shrub isn't very common but, with its tiny lavender flowers and woolly gray foliage, is always enjoyable when found. This shrub can grow up to 10 feet (3 m) tall and 8 feet (2.4 m) wide but is more commonly found smaller in the Sonoran Desert.

Habitat: Mojave and Sonoran Deserts, below 3,000 feet (914 m) in gravelly soils with good drainage.

Blooming season: January through December.

Lifespan: Perrenial, up to twenty years.

Environmental role: Desert lavender blooms often throughout the year, making it a vital nectar source for bees and butterflies. It has a potent scent which also deters pests. It is drought tolerant, making it great for landscaping and promoting biodiversity. It has many medicinal applications for humans as well.

Foraging: The entire desert lavender plant has strong antimicrobial and anti-inflammatory properties. It can be extracted into oils or salves and used topically to treat a variety of conditions from burns and cuts to redness and other skin irritations. It can be used internally in a tincture or tea to treat asthma, allergies, congestion, and lung issues. Its benefits are endless, though not widely studied. Forage in areas where there are more than one bush and only take small amounts from each bush.

Plant friends: Any plant in the mint family (Lamiaceae).

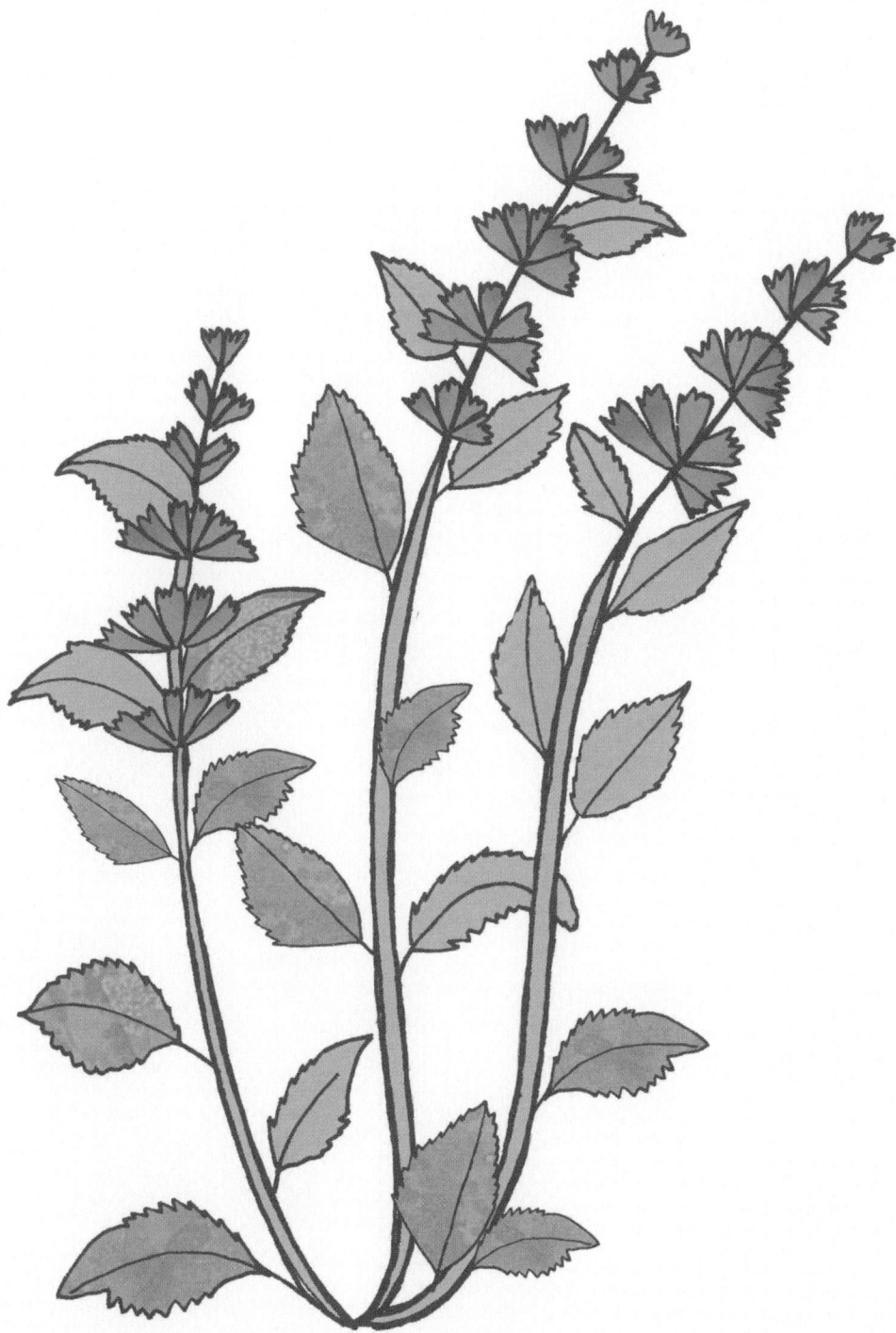

Desert Globemallow

Sphaeralcea ambigua

Appearance: This beloved desert wildflower grows in spikes that cluster at the ground. The small flower heads have five petals and range in color from apricot to pink to red. They have hairy stems and leaves, which help the plant retain water, and their gray color reflects sunlight, which cools the plant. These beauties put on a real show during the springtime throughout the Sonoran Desert and can be found growing alongside showy brittlebush. It can grow up to 3 feet (91 cm) tall and 2 to 3 feet (61 to 91 cm) wide. This is one of my favorite desert wildflowers because of its abundance in the spring.

Habitat: Mojave and Sonoran Deserts below 4,000 feet (1,219 m), in sand, gravel, or rock.

Blooming season: Most abundantly in the spring, though it blooms February through November.

Lifespan: Perennial with a rapid growth rate; can live a little over two years.

Environmental roles: Provides food forage for mule deer, tortoises, bighorn sheep, and cattle. It is important for pollinators, especially bees like the tiny globemallow bee, as it produces many flowers. This plant can colonize soil that has been disturbed by humans or nature, which helps restore native biodiversity and makes it great for desert landscaping.

Foraging: Desert globemallow has long been used by Indigenous peoples in the area for a variety of ailments. It is great as a poultice for cuts, burns, and snake bites, to help encourage healing and reduce swelling. It is great as a tea (strained well) for sore throats and upset stomachs, and to help hydrate via the mucilage it produces (a sticky substance that helps plants retain water). Desert globemallow makes a beautiful addition to spring bouquets as well.

Plant friends: Emory's globemallow, gray globemallow.

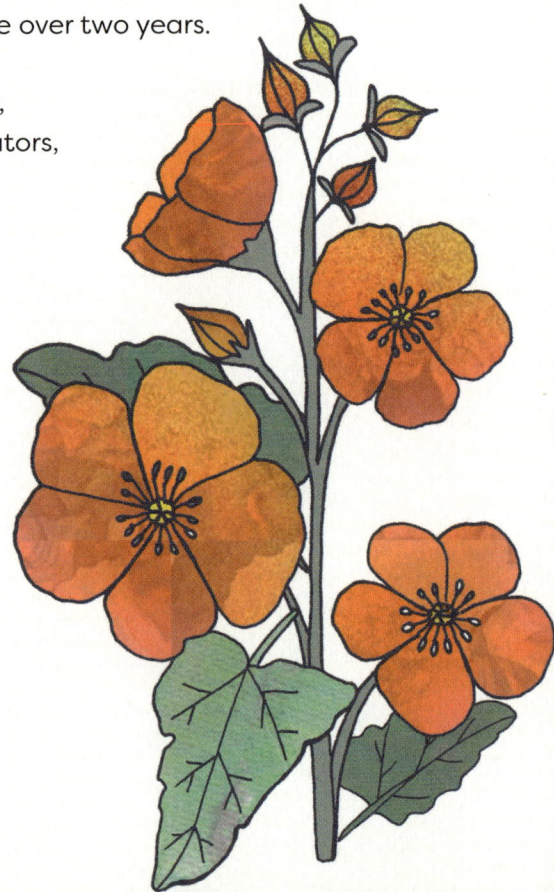

Globemallow Poultice

For cuts, burns, swelling, or slight skin infections. I have personally seen mild infections from a wound of mine heal very quickly using this method, but I am not a doctor or a professional. Try at your own risk.

MATERIALS

- A few large globemallow leaves
- Mortar and pestle
- Rag or washcloth
- Warm water (enough to soak the rag)

INSTRUCTIONS

1. Rinse the globemallow leaves well.

2. Using the mortar and pestle, smash the leaves until wet to create a poultice.

3. Soak the rag in the warm water (hot enough to stand on your skin but not too hot).

4. Apply the poultice directly onto the affected area of skin, then place the warm rag over it. Hold it there until the rag becomes cold, then rewet the rag with warm water and repeat for about 30 minutes.

5. Repeat Step 4 twice daily until the skin issue is healed.

Desert Ironwood Tree

Olneya tesota

Appearance: Desert ironwood is a steadfast desert tree, growing up to 35 feet (11 m) tall. It has dense, thick wood—thus its name. It has small bluish-green leaves that grow in pairs, with a pair of spines located beneath each leaf. In late spring, it loses its leaves and grows striking pinkish-purple flowers all over, creating a beautiful display for a short period. Those flowers then turn into brown seedpods.

Habitat: The Sonoran Desert.

Blooming season: May through June.

Lifespan: Can live up to 800 years!

Environmental roles: Ironwood is ecologically vital because it plays different roles for over 500 species of plants and animals in the Sonoran Desert. It is known as a nurse plant because more than 230 plant species have been found starting their growth under the safety of ironwood trees, including saguaros. Ironwood has also been used in Indigenous cultures for thousands of years. Its shade offers humans and wildlife respite from the hot desert sun, where it can be up to ten degrees cooler under a tree. Wildlife consume its seeds, and pollinators benefit from its flowers.

Foraging: The seeds and flowers of the ironwood tree are edible. The wood from an ironwood is very dense, making it ideal for woodworking, shelter, and charcoal. These trees are truly unique and offer many resources.

Plant friends: Plants in the legume family (Fabaceae).

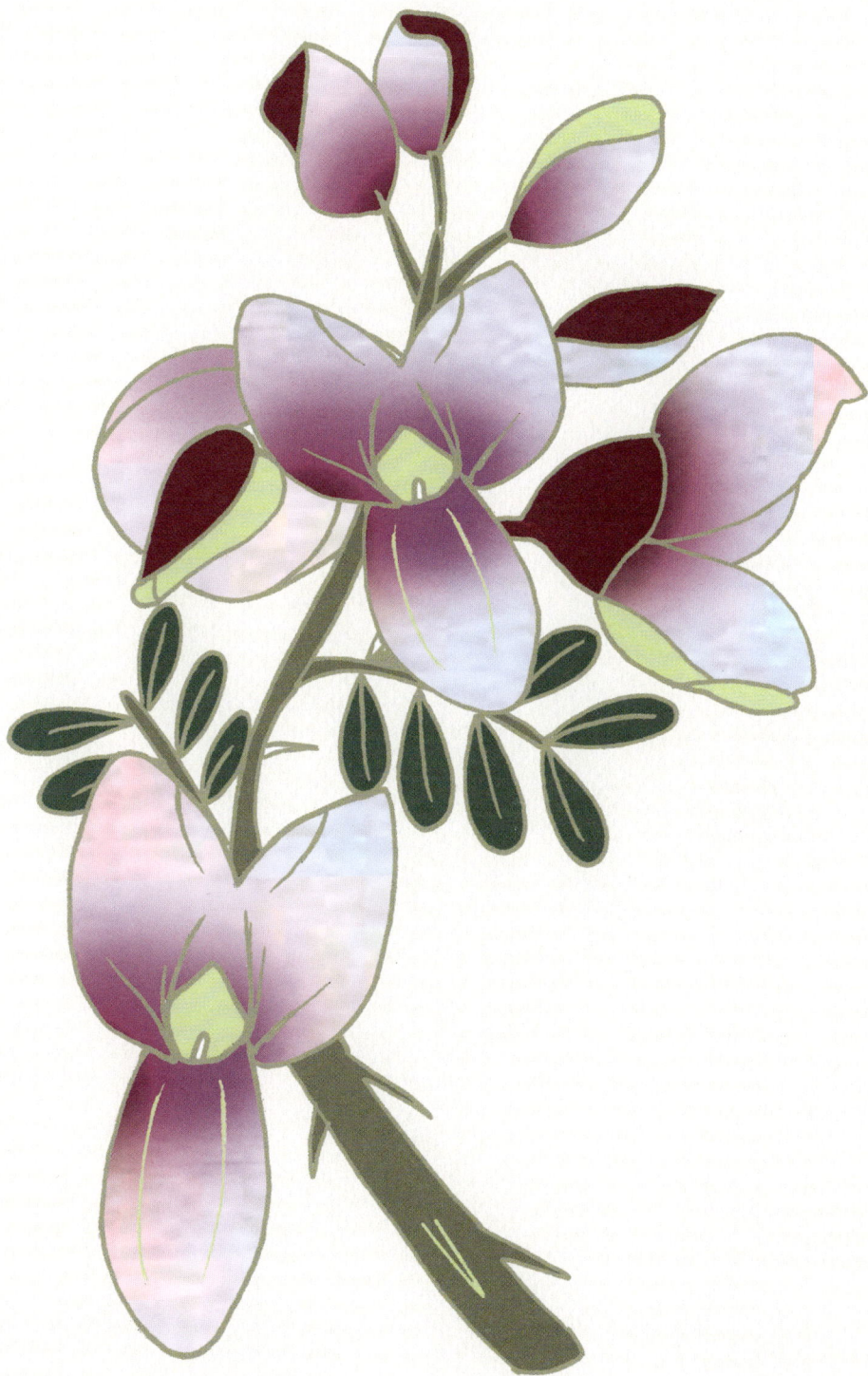

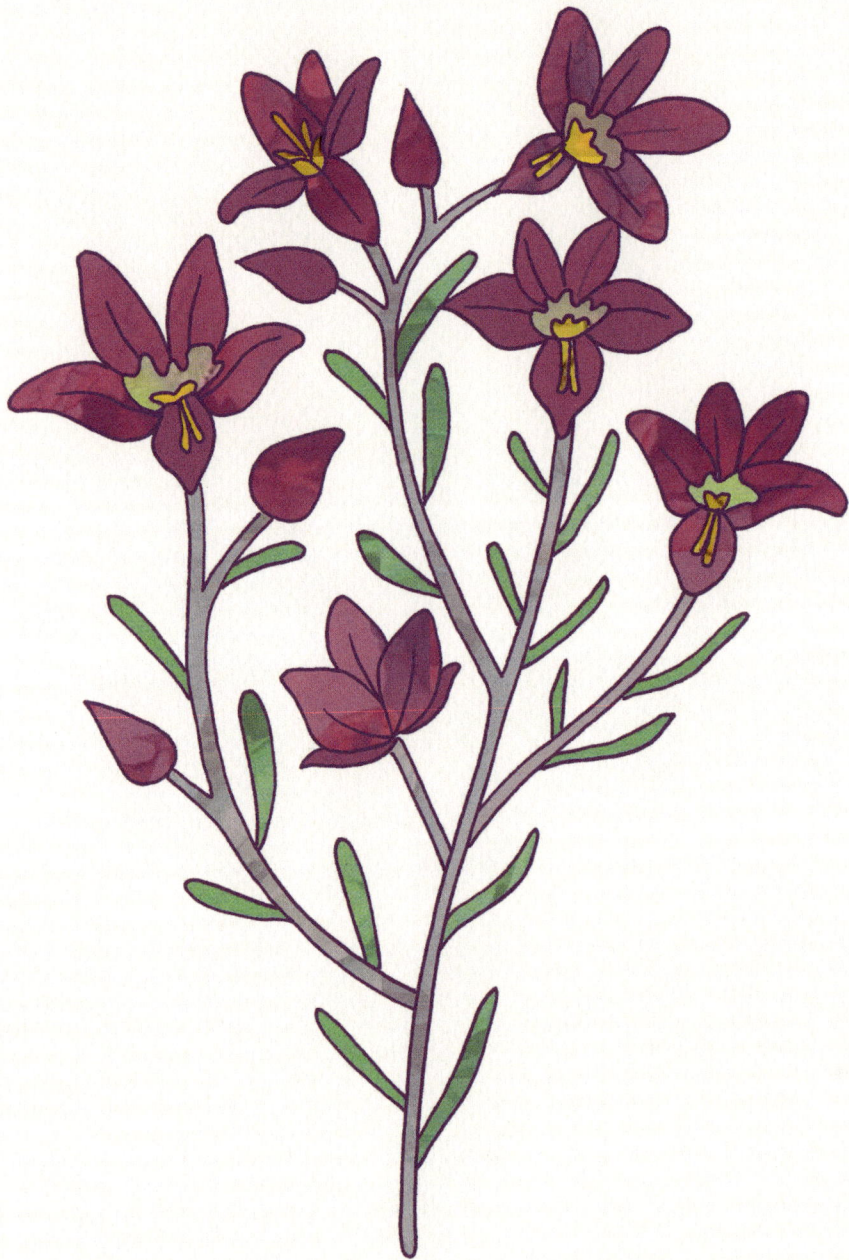

Littleleaf Rhatany

Krameria erecta

Appearance: This pointy subshrub can grow up to 3 feet (91 cm) tall. It has an entanglement of twiggy branches that come to a sharp point. It also has small magenta flowers.

Habitat: The Mojave and Sonoran Deserts, at elevations up to 5,000 feet (1,524 m) on dry, rocky slopes and ridges. They are commonly found growing among creosote bushes.

Blooming season: April through October.

Lifespan: Perennial.

Environmental roles: Littleleaf rhatany can survive very dry conditions because it takes water and nutrients from surrounding plants. Littleleaf rhatany provides oils, not pollen, to visiting female bees, which the bees then feed to their larvae.

Foraging: Native Papago people used the roots to create a red dye to use as ink and to dye textiles, and they also used an infusion of the twigs to treat dysentery and sore eyes. This plant has many possibilities, though more research is needed.

Plant friends: White rhatany.

Desert Mormon Tea

Ephedra fasciculata

Appearance: Desert Mormon tea is one of the many plants in the Ephedra family. This is a small shrub, growing up to 5 feet (1.5 m) tall, with pale-green twigs that turn yellow over time. Each twig is separated into sections by horizontal grooves, creating jointed stems. Each twig produces cones instead of flowers, with the male cones turning light yellow and the female cones turning light brown to green. This plant tends to blend in with the other shrubs and trees of the desert that have similar spiky stems.

Habitat: California, Arizona, Nevada, and southern Utah, on rocky slopes and washes at elevations under 5,000 feet (1,524 m).

Blooming season: Desert Mormon teas do not bloom every year but those that do show their fullest cones in late spring.

Lifespan: Perennial and can live indefinitely. It is a slow-growing plant.

Environmental roles: Desert Mormon tea can conserve water and withstand harsh environments. Wildlife consumes its berries, and the plant also provides shelter for small desert animals. It helps stabilize soil and prevent erosion.

Foraging: This plant is known for its energizing, almost stimulant-like effects. Though, I personally will chew on a stem while I hike through the desert and haven't noticed a huge difference—just a little extra pep. Mormon tea can help with asthma, sinus issues, colds, and coughs, and it can suppress appetites. It can easily be made into a tincture.

Plant friends: Mormon tea and other Ephedra.

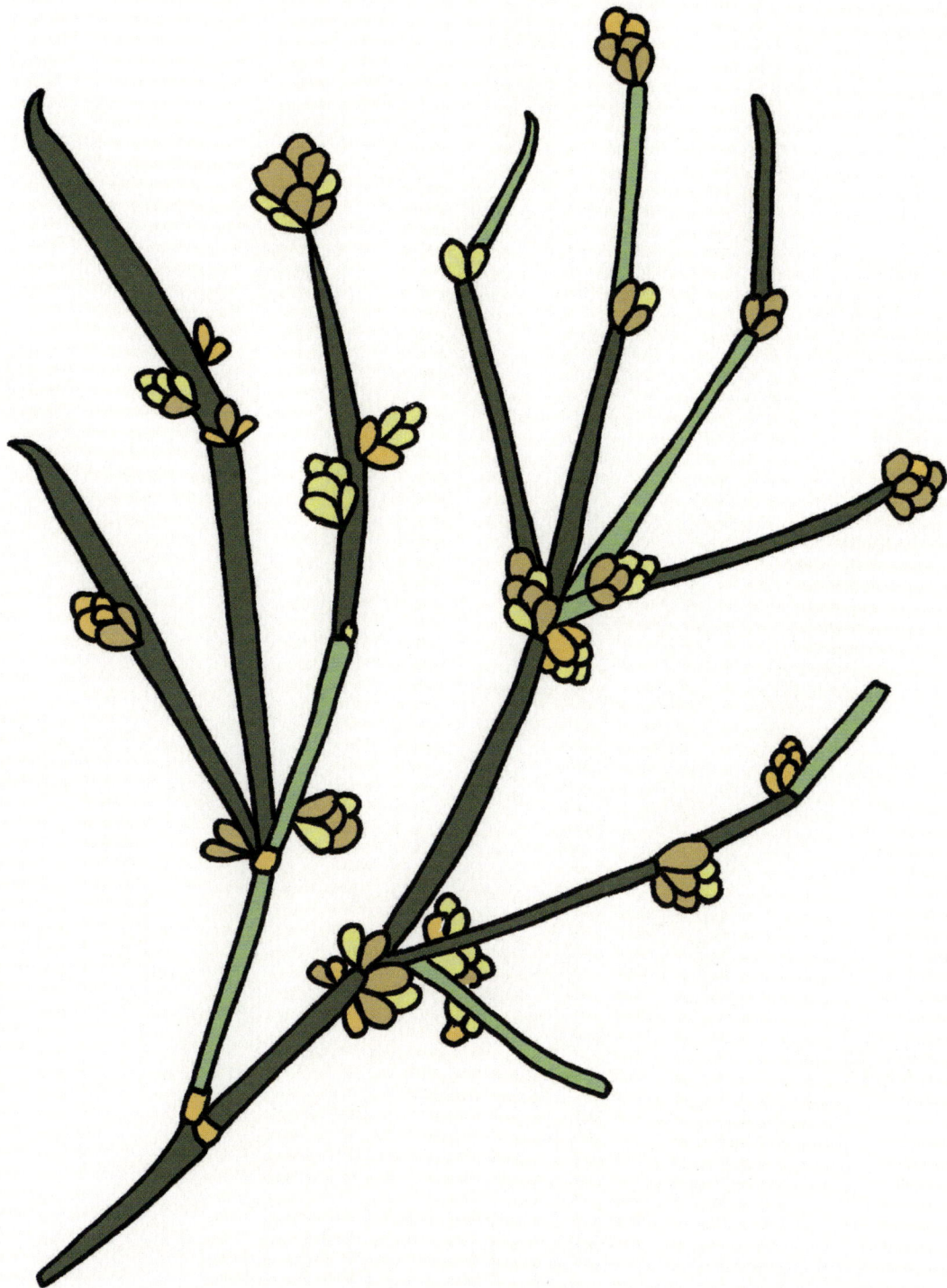

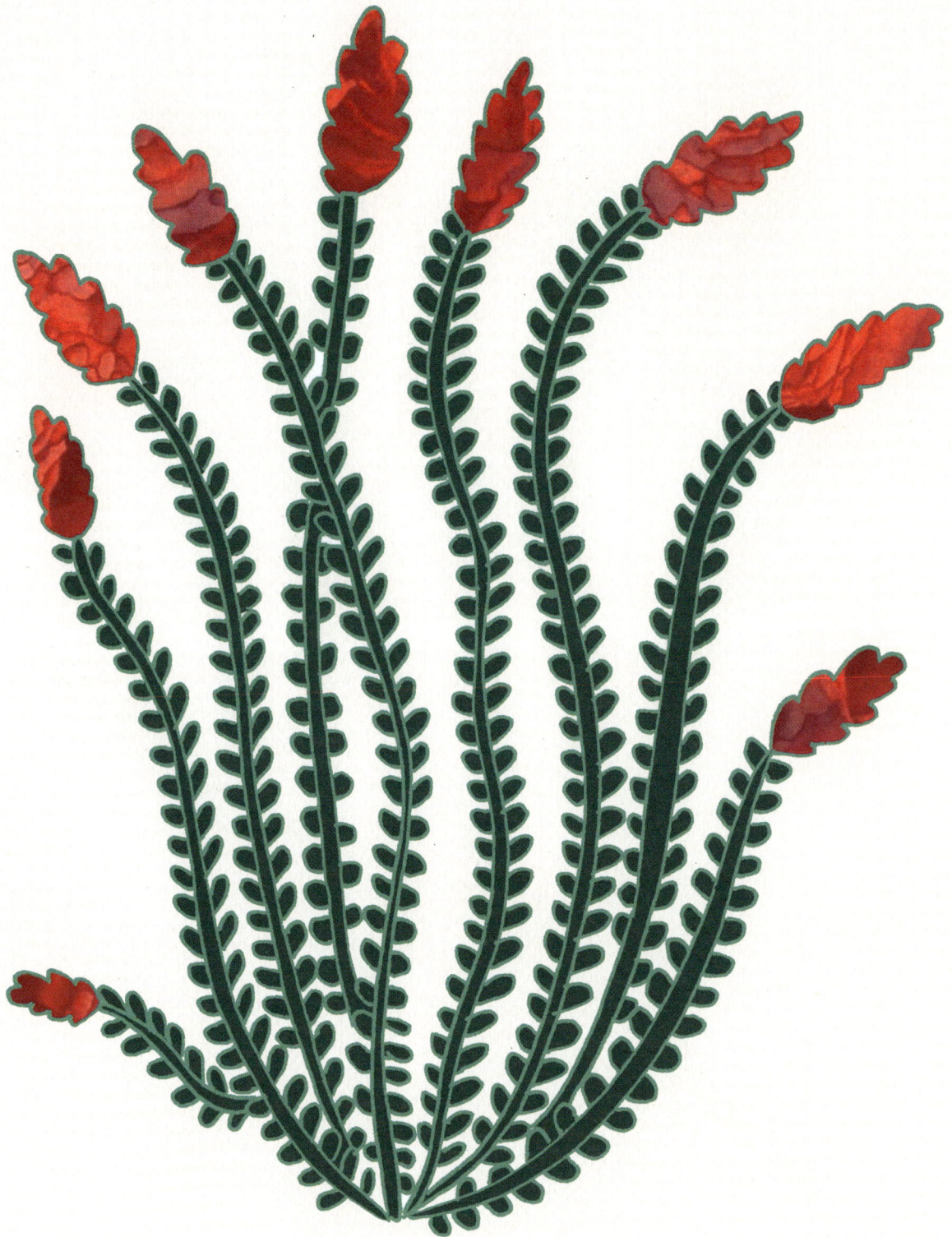

Ocotillo

Fouquieria splendens

Appearance: Ocotillo is a quintessential Sonoran Desert plant. It has a unique look, almost a blend between a tree and a cactus. They are large scrubs with long, cane-like, unbranched, spiny stems. They produce small, 2-inch (5 cm), bright-green oval leaves only after ample rainfall, which drop off during drier months. They are probably best known for their fiery, bright-red, tubular, succulent-like flowers that grow in clusters at the very tip of each long stem.

Habitat: Sonoran and Chihuahuan Deserts in open desert grasslands in rocky, well-draining soil. Ocotillo usually grows in clusters—where you find one in the wild, you will most likely see more.

Blooming season: March through June.

Lifespan: Can live up to one hundred years.

Environmental roles: Ocotillo flowers are a significant source of nectar for native bees and hummingbirds. Ocotillo requires very little water—just 5 to 8 inches (13 to 20 cm) of rain per year—and helps prevent soil erosion.

Foraging: Many people use ocotillo (either dead stems or full, live plants) as fencing because their spines keep people and animals out. I love the way this looks, and it lasts for a long time. Indigenous peoples have used the whole plant medicinally for centuries. The flowers and leaves can be made into a tea or tincture that can help coughs and colds, as well as offering the body extra hydration. The bark can be used in extracts to move the lymph system and the blood, and to support the liver. Its leaves can be made into a poultice for wounds, bruises, and inflamed areas. It is most definitely a very useful desert plant!

Plant friends: Fouquieria is a genus of eleven species of desert flowering plants, making ocotillo very unique. Mexican tree ocotillo is one of its closest relatives.

Yellow Palo Verde & Blue Palo Verde

Parkinsonia microphylla & Parkinsonia florida

Appearance: Both these trees are Sonoran Desert mainstays. They range in size from 15 to 30 feet (4.5 to 9 m) tall. The phrase palo verde means "green stick." The yellow palo verde has bright-green bark, while the blue palo verde's bark has more of a blue-green color. They both have bright-yellow flowers, with those of the blue palo verde being slightly brighter. When they bloom, their flowers cover the entire canopy of its branches, making for a striking display throughout the desert. They both also have small leaves and small thorns.

Habitat: The Sonoran Desert, up to an elevation of 5,000 feet (1,524 m). Yellow palo verde trees require less water, so they can be found in higher upland areas, where the soil is coarser (meaning it retains less water), and blue palo verde can be found mostly in or near washes.

Blooming season: Blue palo verde blooms first in March and April, while the yellow palo verde blooms later in April and in May.

Lifespan: Perennial, with a potential lifespan up to four hundred years.

Environmental roles: Palo verdes are the primary nurse plant for saguaros. They are an important food source for wildlife and humans alike. They offer shade from the hot desert sun, cooling the areas where they grow. Their flowers are an extremely important nectar source for desert pollinators, because they produce so many flowers continuously throughout the spring. Their seeds are a food source for desert wildlife and for humans. All desert trees help stabilize the ecosystem and are vital to its health.

Foraging: The flowers and seeds from palo verde pods are edible. I like to forage the flowers to eat with salads, as they have a distinct tangy flavor. The seeds can be dried and turned into flour or can be eaten fresh (I prefer them fresh). The fresh seeds have the texture of edamame and can be used in a variety of recipes or eaten alone. They are a great source of protein.

Plant friend: Jerusalem thorn and velvet mesquite.

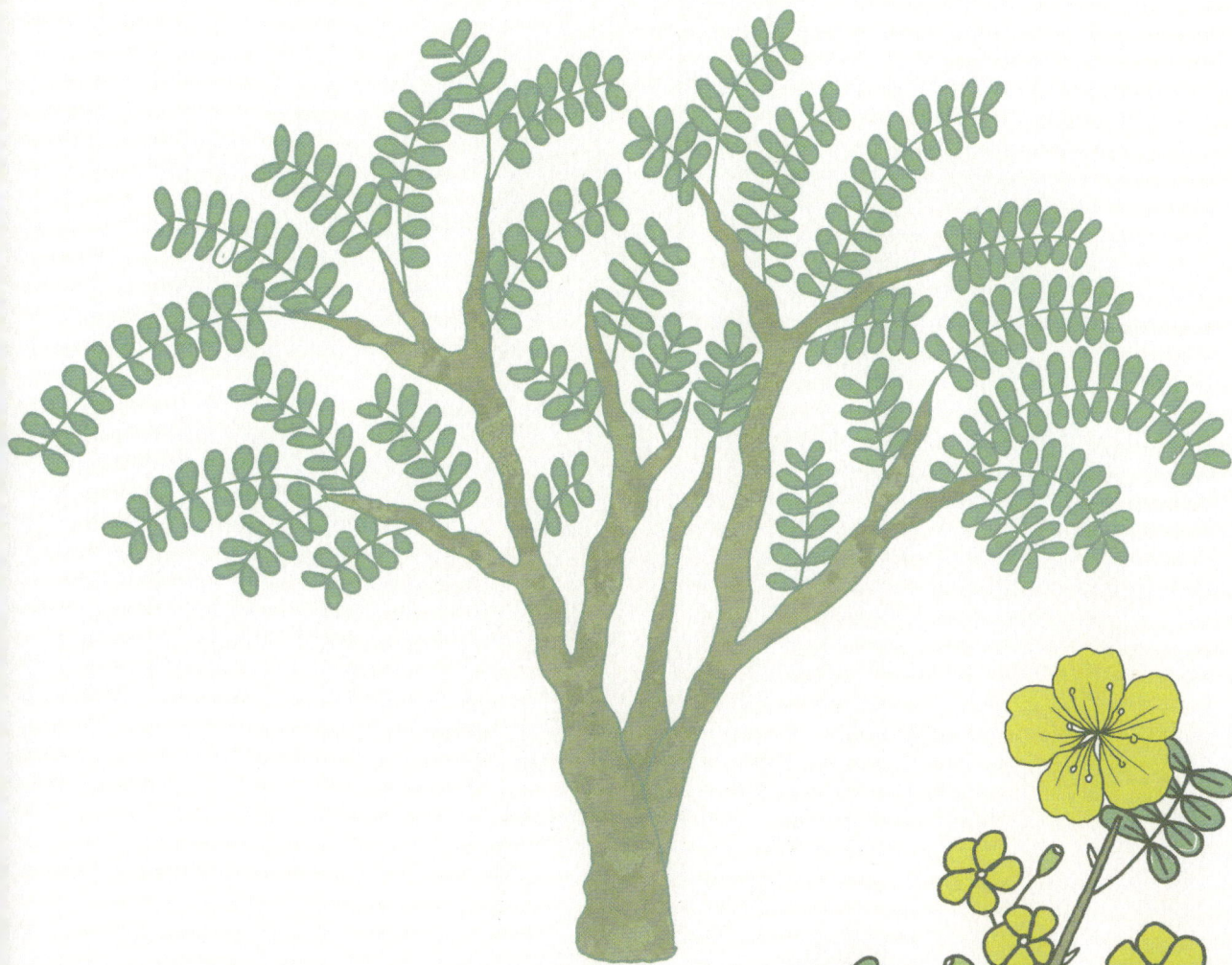

Blue Palo Verde

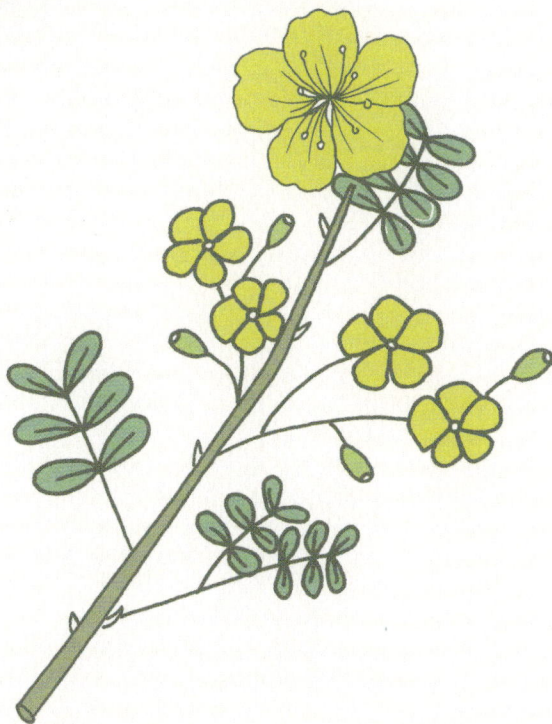

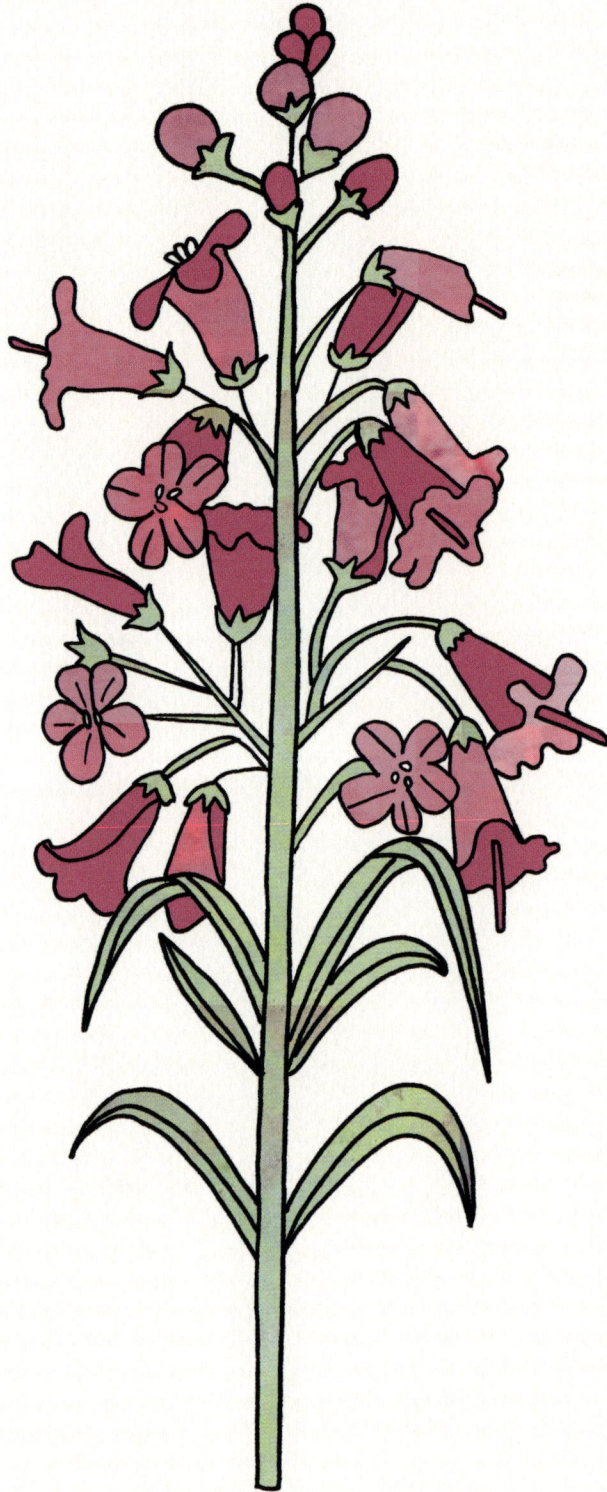

Parry's Penstemon

Penstemon parryi

Appearance: Parry's penstemon is a truly gorgeous desert wildflower. It grows erect, about 1 to 5 feet (0.3 to 1.5 m) tall, with long, thick, blue-green, lance-shaped leaves. Many tubular bright-pink flowers form at the ends of the stems in a spike formation. They mimic succulents with their waxy coating. These fast-growing flowers are so inviting, like bright little flagpoles on the desert floor.

Habitat: The Sonoran Desert, in mountain canyons, desert washes, and grassland slopes.

Blooming season: March through May.

Lifespan: Three to five years. They die when the summer heat sets in, but their tiny seeds spread so easily, they will often sprout new plants in the same area.

Environmental roles: Parry's penstemon offers rich nectar to a wide range of desert pollinators. They are drought-tolerant and fast-growing, so they're great for large-scale revegetation and erosion control projects. They are a spring staple here in the desert.

Foraging: I love to collect these for fresh wildflower bouquets because they last quite a while in a water-filled vase. Their bright-pink color adds a unique shade to desert-wildflower bouquets, as it stands out among the yellows and oranges of many of the other wildflowers.

Plant friends: Firecracker penstemon, Palmer's penstemon.

Santa Rita Prickly Pear Cactus

Opuntia santa-rita

Appearance: The Santa Rita prickly pear is striking, with pads that range in color from bluish green to pink to bright purple. They can grow up to 8 feet (2.4 m) tall and 10 feet (3 m) wide, with many pads on a few main stalks. The cactus pads have no spines, but they have tons of tiny glochids. Large, bright-yellow, waxy flowers 3 to 5 inches (7.5 to 13 cm) in diameter bloom along the edges of the pads. These flowers then grow into small fruits.

Habitat: Sonoran and Chihuahuan Deserts, and Baja California, growing in sandy or gravelly soil.

Blooming season: April through June, blooming over and over again until the heat comes.

Lifespan: Perennial, up to thirty years.

Environmental roles: Prickly pear cacti are vital for native bees as a source of pollen and a safe place to rest. The flowers close as the sun starts to set and open again in the morning, so bees can sleep inside the flowers overnight. Prickly pear cactus fruits are an important food source for wildlife, rich in electrolytes and vitamins. These cacti also provide shelter for birds, reptiles, and rodents. They can also mediate contaminated soil, making for cleaner environments.

Foraging: The fruits of this cactus are edible, but small and not very juicy; I tend not to harvest them. They propagate very easily. I remove a pad carefully with tongs (careful not to touch the cactus at all as it has glochids that can irritate the skin), let it dry for a day or two, and then just stick it in the dirt, where it will grow an entirely new plant from just one pad.

Plant friends: Engelman's prickly pear cactus and all other *Opuntia* cactus.

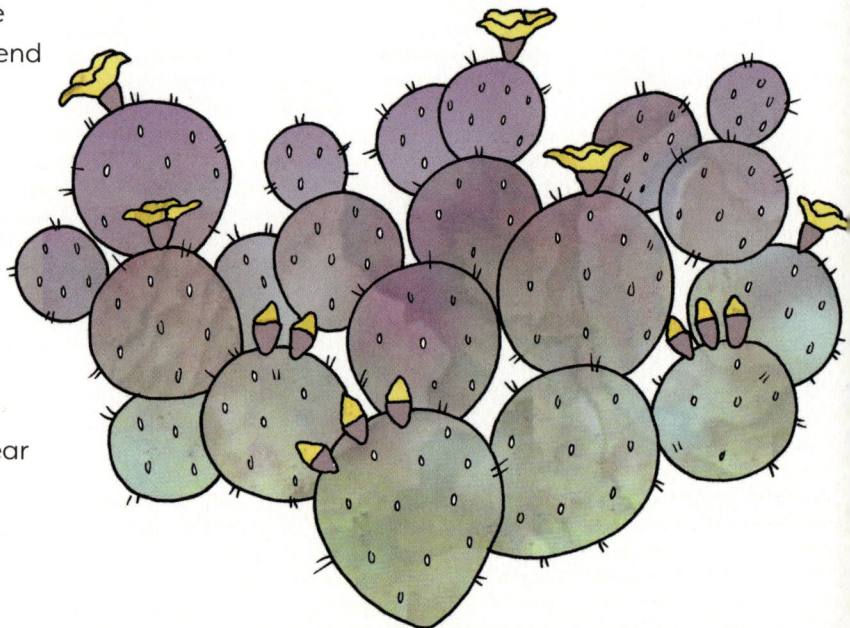

Harvesting and Dyeing with Cochineal

Learn how to create an all-natural (non-vegan) dye from foraged cochineal! Cochineal is a mealy bug that tends to grow on prickly pear cacti here in the Sonoran Desert. They produce a sticky, fluffy white material that protects them from being eaten by birds. They are parasitic to the prickly pear, sucking nutrients directly from the cactus. They tend to thrive on weakened or sickly cacti. I harvest these bugs to dye textiles like cotton and linen.

MATERIALS

- Jar or large yogurt container
- Large metal spoon
- Distilled water (the amount will vary depending on how much cochineal you collect)
- Pestle
- Mordanted fabric
- Large pot (big enough to soak the fabric)
- Water, to fill the pot
- Fine-mesh strainer

➤ *This all-natural dye creates a beautiful, long-lasting pink or magenta on natural fabrics. Other techniques can create colors like purple and red. To preserve the color of the dye, it's best to hand-wash and line-dry the dyed fabric.*

INSTRUCTIONS

1. Scrape the white fluff off the cactus into the jar with the large metal spoon. You will see the red smears of the bugs (that is the dye produced by the cochineal, called carmine). Collect a decent amount. (You can play around with the amount, depending on how dark you want the color to turn out.)

2. Add enough distilled water to cover the cochineal you collected, then crush it with the pestle in the jar; this releases more of the dye.

3. Make a dye bath: fill the large pot with the mordanted fabric you want to dye and cover the cloth with water.

4. Use the fine-mesh strainer to strain the cochineal water mixture (dye) you made in Step 2 into the dye bath.

5. Repeat Step 2 a few times, continually adding the dye to the dye bath, until the cochineal's color has faded.

6. Let the cloth sit in the dye bath for 8 to 24 hours. Remove the cloth and rinse well with cold water.

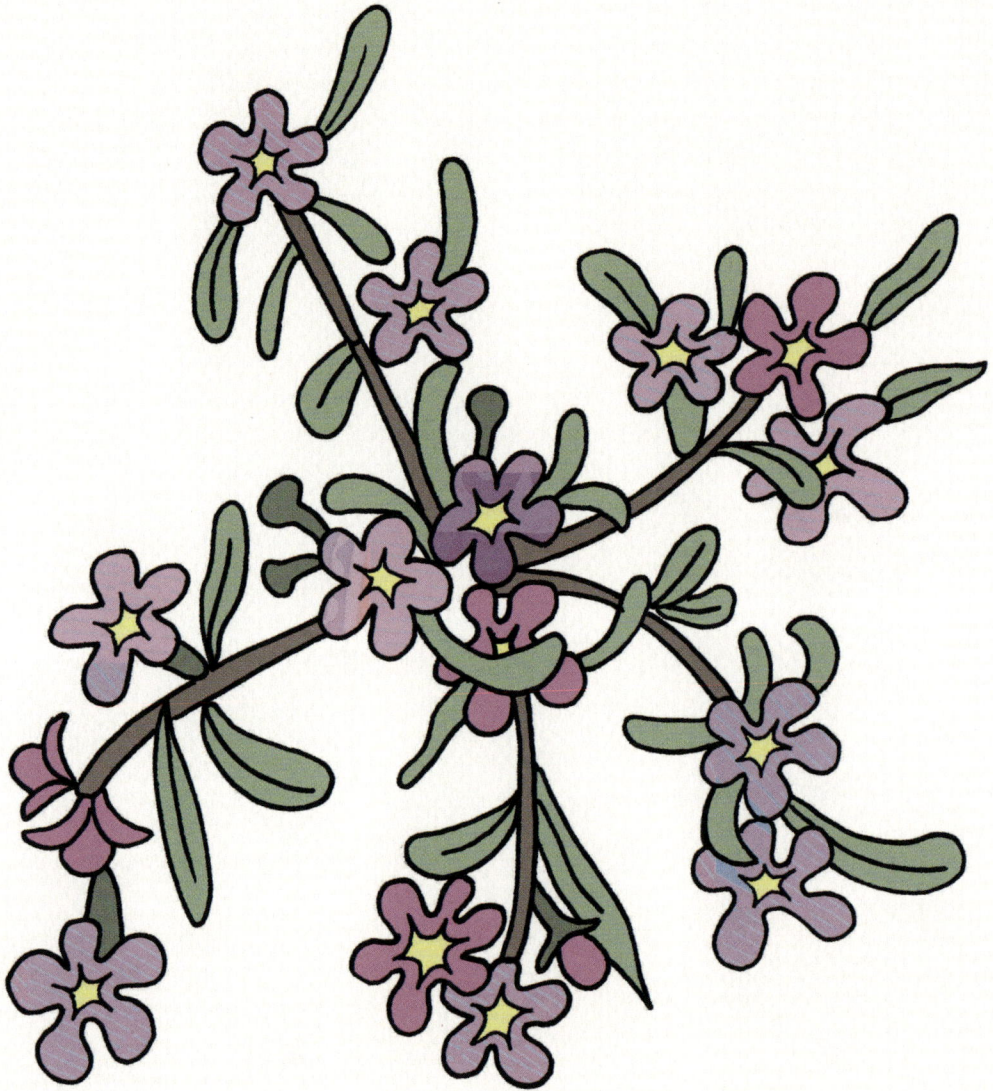

Purple Mat

Nama demissum

Appearance: This vibrant, small, low-growing plant spreads over the desert floor and can grow up to 8 inches (20 cm) long and only a couple of inches tall. It has slender, hairy stems with several small, bell-shaped, purplish flowers.

Habitat: *Nama* in Greek means "a water spring." This plant can be found after adequate rainfall and near desert washes in the Sonoran Desert.

Blooming season: February through July.

Lifespan: Annual. Sprouts after adequate winter rains and dies off in the peak of the summer heat.

Environmental roles: Purple mat plays a vital role in the ecosystem. It creates important ground cover by forming "mats" on the desert floor that help stabilize and maintain moisture in the soil and reduce erosion. They are hardy plants that can survive freezing temperatures at night and over 100°F (38°C) during the day. Their flowers are also important for pollinators.

Foraging: No known direct uses for humans.

Plant friends: Sand bells.

Saguaro

Carnegiea gigantea

Appearance: The saguaro cactus is the icon of the Sonoran Desert and what people usually think of when they think of desert plants. This impressive plant is the largest cactus in the United States, growing up to 50 feet (15 m) tall! Saguaros are often seen as the wise, ancient ones, guarding the desert. They have a thick, spine-protected trunk that is well-adapted to swell and shrink depending on rainfall. Its well-known upturned arms start to develop after seventy-five years of growth. In the spring, saguaros produce large, waxy, whitish-yellow flowers, usually at the tips of their arms. Saguaros in bloom are one of my favorite springtime experiences.

Habitat: Exclusively in the Sonoran Desert, mostly in southern Arizona and western Sonora, Mexico. Live between sea level and up to 4,500 feet (1,372 m).

Blooming season: End of April through the first week of June.

Lifespan: This slow-growing cactus can live up to two hundred years.

Environmental roles: The saguaro is a keystone species, meaning that other species in the ecosystem depend on it. It provides food, shelter, nesting sites, and nectar to desert wildlife. Its large root system helps transmute nitrogen into a form that animals can use and also helps tremendously with soil erosion.

Foraging: Saguaro flowers should not be foraged because they turn into vital fruit in the summer (see page 88). Dried saguaro ribs (the long, woody, skeleton pieces from a dead saguaro) are useful for creating shelter, fencing, and other decorative items.

Plant friends: Saguaros are the only plant in the *Carnegiea* genus, but they are related to all other cacti in the Cactaceae family, like the barrel cactus and the cardon cactus.

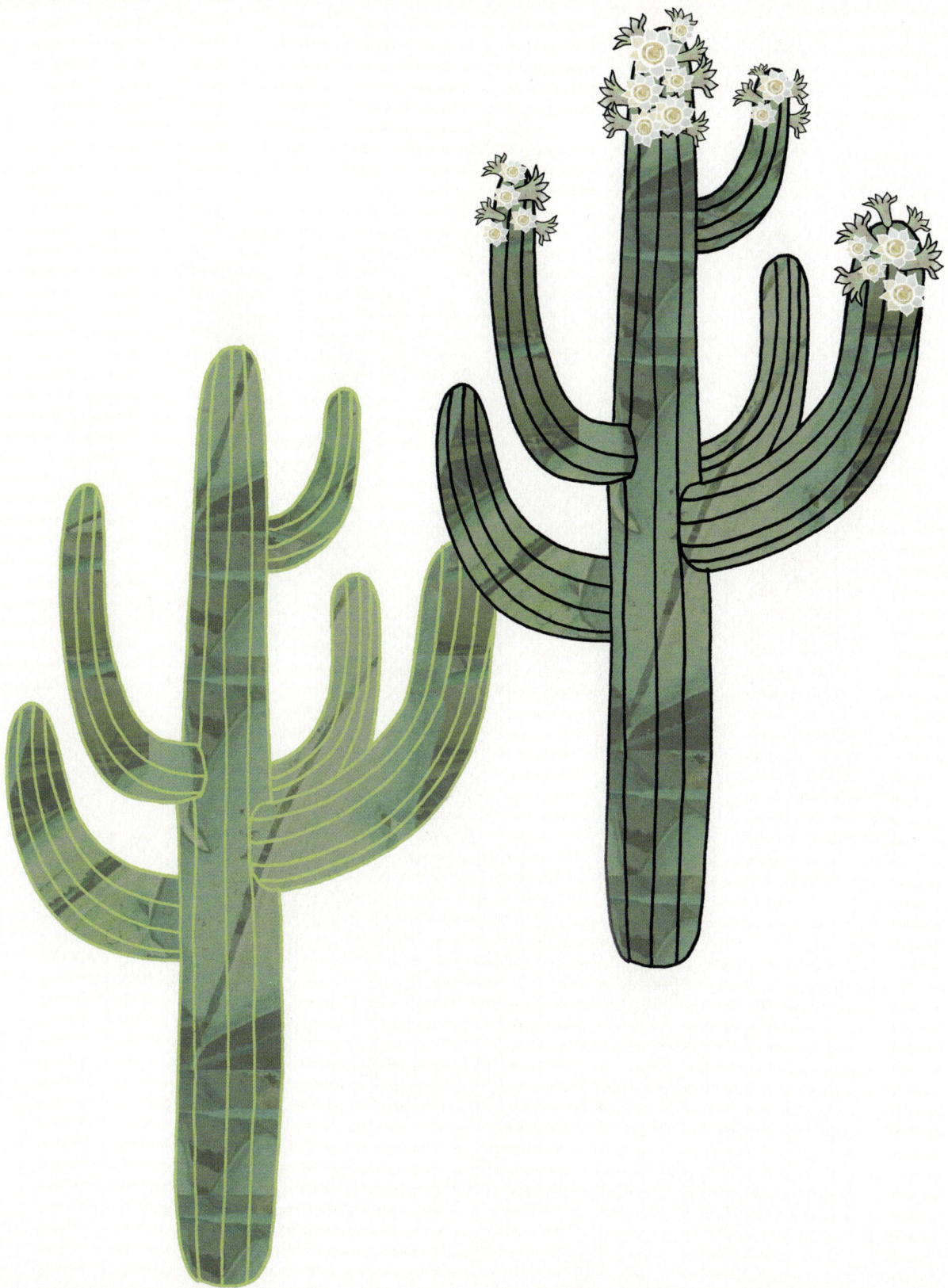

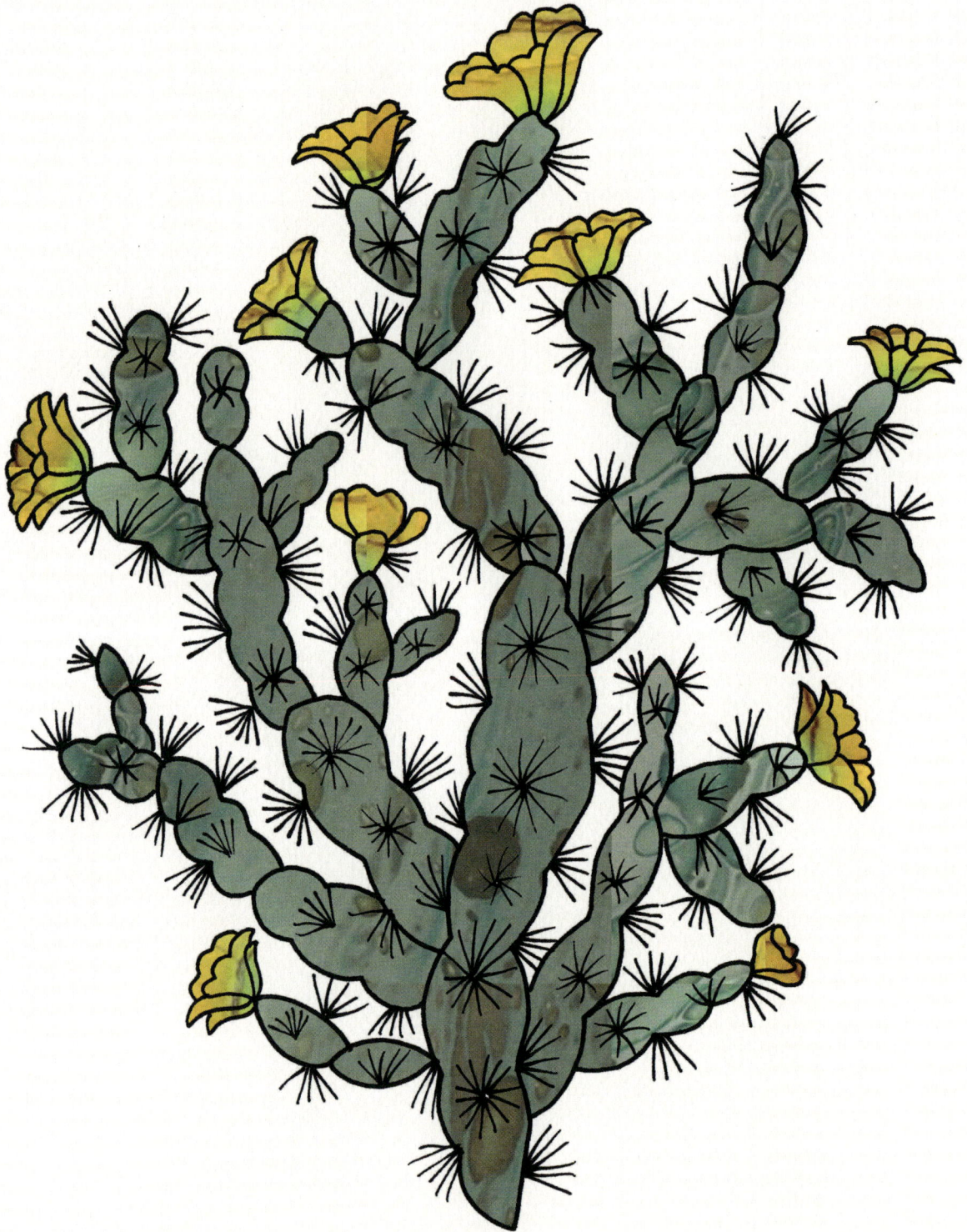

Staghorn Cholla

Cylindropuntia versicolor

Appearance: This cactus is unique, with its slender green to purple stems. It grows in an upright branched formation up to 6 feet (1.8 m) tall, with shorter, bristlelike spines. And those spines definitely hurt! Staghorn cholla is best known for its brilliant flower display. Even two of these cacti next to each other can have two different colors of flower, including red, orange, yellow, purple, and magenta. The flowers usually form on the end of a stem and form small green fruits that eventually turn yellow to red.

Habitat: Only grows in southern Arizona and northern Mexico in scrubland and grassland between 2,000 and 4,000 feet (610 and 1,219 m).

Blooming season: April to June.

Lifespan: Thirty or more years, and can easily propagate when a stem is detached and falls onto a suitable area where it can grow roots easily.

Environmental roles: Cholla's spiny branches provide shelter for many desert animals, protecting them from predators. The cholla's fruit is a vital food source for javelina, deer, and bighorn sheep. The cholla flowers give pollen to bees and nectar to hummingbirds. Native bees often sleep in the cholla flowers, as the flowers close in the evening and open with the sun.

Foraging: Cholla are most known for their edible flower buds, which offer hydration and are high in calcium. The buds are picked just before they open, and then de-thorned, cooked, and eaten or dried for later use. If foraging for cholla buds, be sure to leave the majority of the buds for the flowers to bloom, and be sure to use tongs when removing from the cactus.

Plant friends: Buckhorn cholla (very similar), teddy bear cholla, chain fruit cholla, and other *Cylindropuntia.*

Summer

Here Comes the Rain

June through August

Summer in the Sonoran Desert sweeps in fast. Spring wildflowers crisp up, and the heat glistens on the horizon as desert temperatures rise. Still, even without rain, mesquites leaf out and seed and giant saguaros set bright-red crowns of fruit, sweet and full of electrolytes. These plants sustain all desert dwellers, from the small millipede to the lumbering human. As the days get longer and hotter, watering holes dry up, plants drop their leaves, and animals retreat to shade or underground. In July, dark clouds begin to build and, after weeks of anticipation, lightning breaks the skies open to release hard rains that permeate the desert floor and fill arroyos in a flash. The monsoons lower the temperature, and all beings celebrate the much-needed respite. The moisture releases oils from the leaves of the creosote bush, and fills the air with a petrichor scent, the nostalgic aroma of Sonoran rain. Shrubbery comes back to life and saguaros plump up as they soak up the rain. The desert is green once again. Summer is a time of both survival and relief, as life slows down during the long days.

A lot of people complain about summer in the Sonoran Desert, because this is the season when temperatures rise drastically. Temperatures average around 104°F (40°C) but often reach 118°F (48°C) in the hotter months, such as June and July. This can make for tough living for us humans, especially in cities where asphalt and concrete rule and cause temperatures to rise even further.

Summer in the Sonoran Desert can be divided into two chunks: June, when the heat is most unbearable and everything has dried up, and then monsoon season in July and August, when we receive most of our yearly rain all in a handful of torrential downpours. Desert monsoons bring lightning storms, dust storms, flash floods, sporadic rain, and even hail! But the monsoon season also brings everything back to life. Temperatures cool down during and after the storms to a cool 78 to 80°F (26 to 27°C), and the potent oils of the creosote bush are released into the air, calming and grounding desert dwellers with its nostalgic scent. The grasslands are especially green and happy during this time, and there is so much food to be found. The toads emerge after the storms for a few nights to mate and eat, and then return underground.

Summer in the desert is a reptile's dream, as they soak up the sun, but those reptiles also make for tasty snacks for roadrunners and hawks. The juxtaposition of the intense heat with the immense rain truly creates a sort of tropical paradise, especially in southern Arizona. Summer is a time of abundance, as the prickly pear fruits ripen, the native edible greens grow in hoards, and mesquite beans start to fall. Time to take stock for the upcoming dry spells of autumn.

Palmer Amaranth

Amaranthus palmeri

Appearance: This hardy, tall-growing pigweed has green, oval- to elliptical-shaped leaves. It grows erect and has one main stem with leaves and branches around it. This plant grows a tall spike at the top with tiny whitish-green flowers that eventually turn into small, millet-like seeds.

Habitat: Grows in lower and upper deserts below 5,500 feet (1,676 m) in the southern United States and northwestern Mexico and in a variety of soil types: riverbeds, fields, roadsides, and irrigated lands. Usually comes up after monsoon rains.

Blooming season: July through late September.

Lifespan: Annual.

Environmental role: Even though this plant is considered a "weed" by most people, it has been and continues to be an important food source for so many animals and humans. Amaranth leaves have tons of minerals and vitamins. The seeds are also highly nutritious, and birds love them. This plant is also thought to have the ability to remove toxins from damaged soil, which is why it is usually the first to grow in areas that have been damaged by human intervention.

Foraging: This plant has been used as a food source by Indigenous peoples in the Southwest for thousands of years. The leaves taste very similar to spinach when cooked and can be used as spinach can in a variety of dishes (see page 57 for recipe).

Plant friends: This plant is in the pigweed family and is related to Hopi red dye amaranth, prostrate pigweed, and fringed pigweed. You'll very often find this plant growing next to types of purslanes.

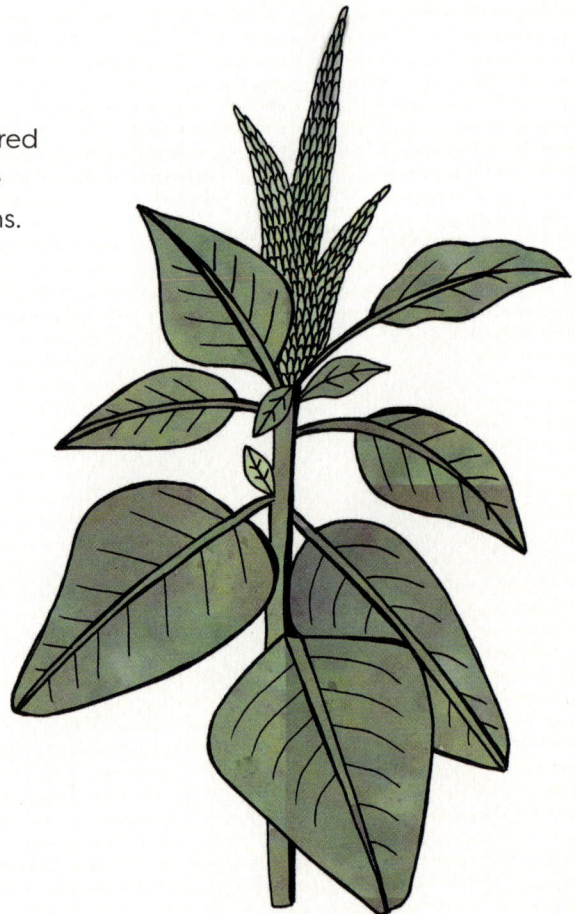

Palmer Amaranth Calabacitas Entrée

Amaranth has been consumed by Indigenous peoples all over the United States for thousands of years. The plant's leaves are free and plentiful during monsoon season here in the desert. They are also high in vitamins like iron and calcium, as well as protein, and could even be growing in your backyard! I have tons of it growing in my backyard and made this delicious meal with it that I would like to share with you. When foraging Palmer amaranth (or any kind of amaranth) for this dish, make sure it's growing in a safe place (away from roadsides).

INGREDIENTS

- 30 to 40 Palmer amaranth leaves (I recommend younger leaves, as they are more tender, less rough, and less bitter. You can feel the difference: the younger leaves feel softer and are a brighter green color)
- Olive oil, for cooking
- 1 ear of corn, kernels cut from the cob
- ½ yellow summer squash, diced
- Tajín, for seasoning
- Cotija cheese, for serving
- Tortillas or sourdough bread, for serving (optional)

INSTRUCTIONS

1. Rinse the amaranth leaves well.

2. Heat a large skillet over medium heat. Pour the olive oil into the skillet and add the corn and squash.

3. Add a few hard shakes of Tajín and stir.

4. Once the corn and squash are almost fully cooked, add the amaranth and stir, cooking until the amaranth is wilted.

5. Add some cotija cheese and enjoy by itself or with a tortilla or sourdough bread.

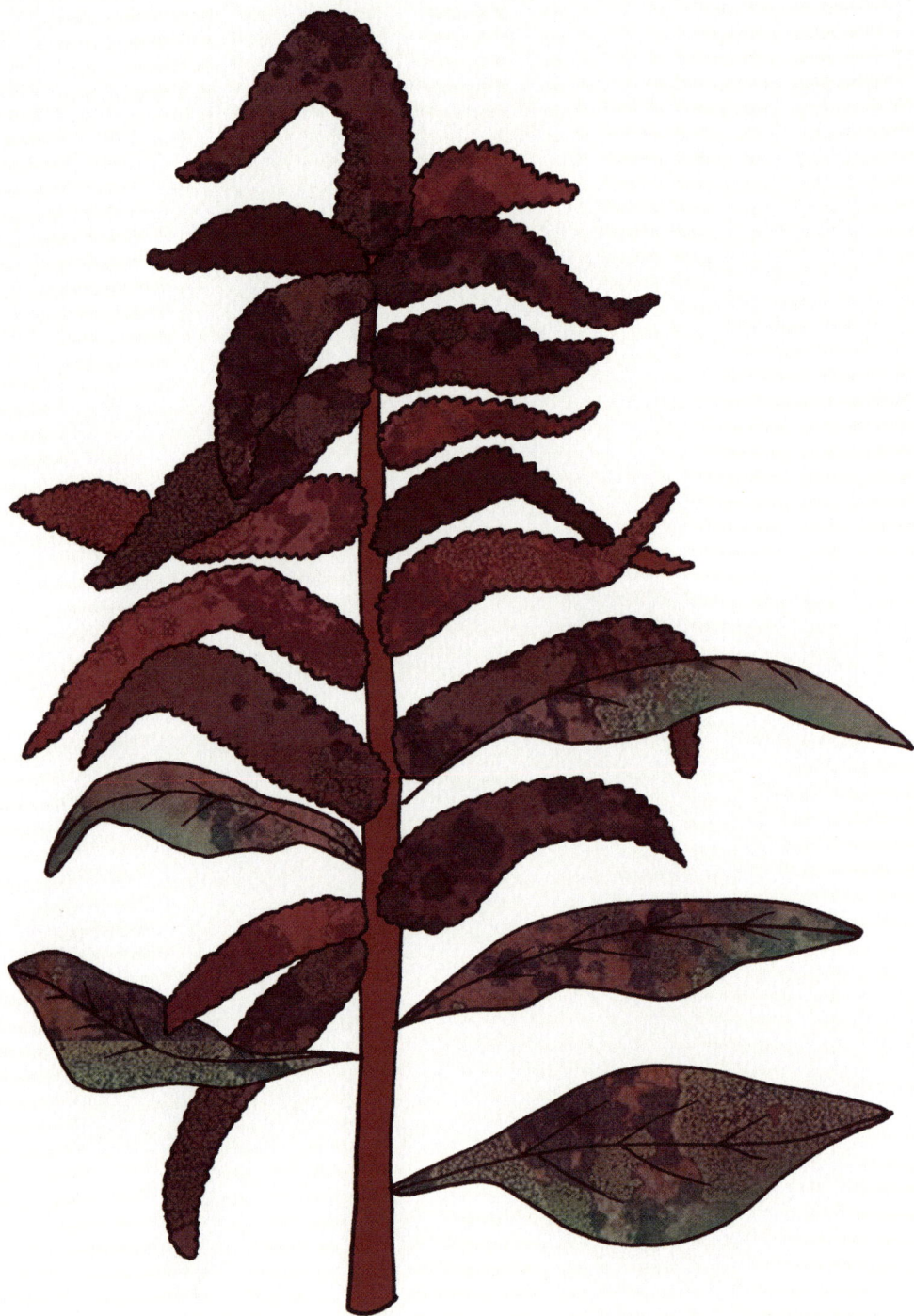

Hopi Red Dye Amaranth

Amaranthus cruentus / Komo (local Hopi name)

Appearance: This gorgeous plant grows erect and has one main stem with leaves and branches around it. The leaves are green with magenta veins. Hopi red dye amaranth grows a tall magenta spike at the top with tiny magenta flowers that eventually turn into small, millet-like seeds.

Habitat: This plant is thought to be native to central Mexico but spread to the Southwestern United States through domestication by Indigenous peoples like the Hopi. There are not too many areas where this specific type of amaranth grows wild as it was domesticated four thousand years ago, but seeds have been collected from the Hopi reservation in Arizona. This plant does well in gardens in Arizona and many other areas of the United States. Although it is rare, it is not considered threatened due to domestication.

Blooming season: July through October.

Lifespan: Annual, but the seeds are plentiful and will survive until the next season in the soil, growing new plants when the time is right.

Environmental roles: Hopi red dye amaranth is a hardy plant that can survive arid conditions and full sun. These plants were vital to the Aztec, who believed they were the food of the gods. The Hopi people generally grow them on irrigated terraces. These plants are great as a food source for humans and wildlife and as a source for a natural, edible dye. The Hopi use the pink dye that is extracted from the flowers to create wafers that are associated with benevolent beings that bring blessings.

Foraging: Hopi red dye amaranth is edible in the same ways other amaranths are. The leaves have great nutritional value and are easily digestible, similar to spinach. The entire plant can be used to extract a pink to magenta dye that can be used for dyeing textiles and can be used to dye foods.

Plant friends: Other pigweeds like Palmer's amaranth and prostrate pigweed.

Arizona Poppy

Kallstroemia grandiflora

Appearance: When summer rain is plentiful, Arizona poppies put on a brilliant show. They resemble California poppies but are not related to poppies and the differences are obvious when closely observed. They grow in clumps spreading over the ground, with each plant growing about 2 to 3 feet (61 to 91 cm) tall. They have long, hairy, thin, trailing stems with bright-orange, five-petal flowers with dark-red centers, about 2½ inches (6 cm) in size. They have leaves that mirror each other, about five to ten 1-inch (2.5 cm) leaflets along each side of the stem. They are my personal favorite summer wildflower—I even named my shop in Tucson after them!

Habitat: Southern Arizona, California, New Mexico, and west Texas, in sandy deserts, grassland plains, and mesas below 3,000 feet (914 m).

Blooming season: June through September.

Lifespan: Annual. They germinate after summer rains and dry out and seed as the season changes to autumn.

Environmental roles: The seeds play an important role as a food source for native birds. Arizona poppies are also often used in desert restoration because they can grow well in disturbed areas. They are food sources for pollinators like butterflies, bees, and hummingbirds. Indigenous peoples used Arizona poppies medicinally. They are often seen growing along roadsides, adding beauty to our city landscape.

Foraging: The Arizona poppy root can be used in a tea to help with stomachaches, diarrhea, and fevers. The tea can also be used after a sprain or bruise to help stabilize the injury and promote healing. Forage responsibly (see the Sustainable Foraging section for help).

Plant friends: Puncture vine is in the caltrop family (the same as Arizona poppy), is invasive in Arizona, and grows a sharp, detachable, thorn-covered head that can be bothersome to humans and animals. Arizona poppy and puncture vine look similar when the plants are young, making Arizona poppies more susceptible to being removed. To tell the difference, note puncture vines' smaller size and smaller yellow flowers.

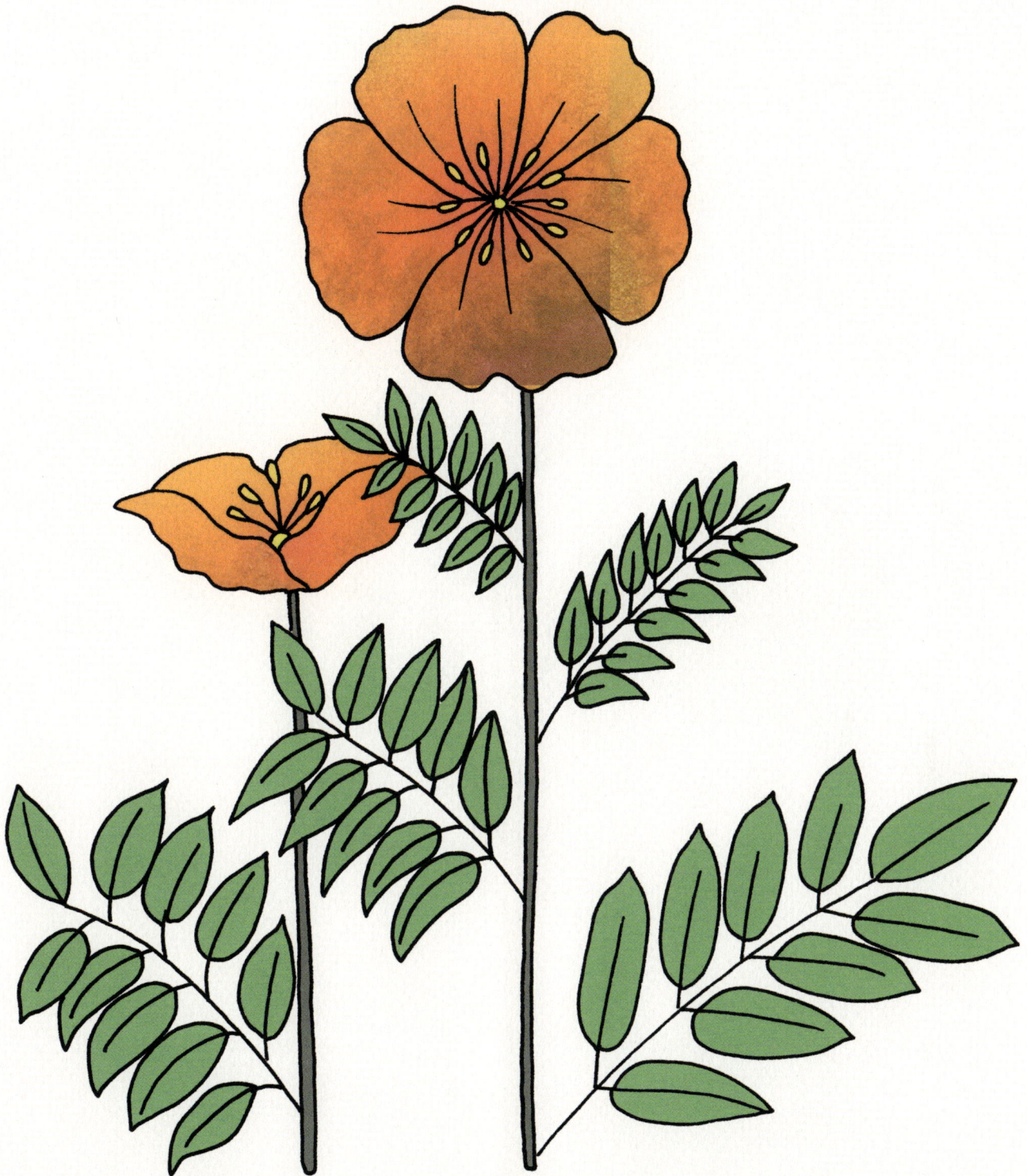

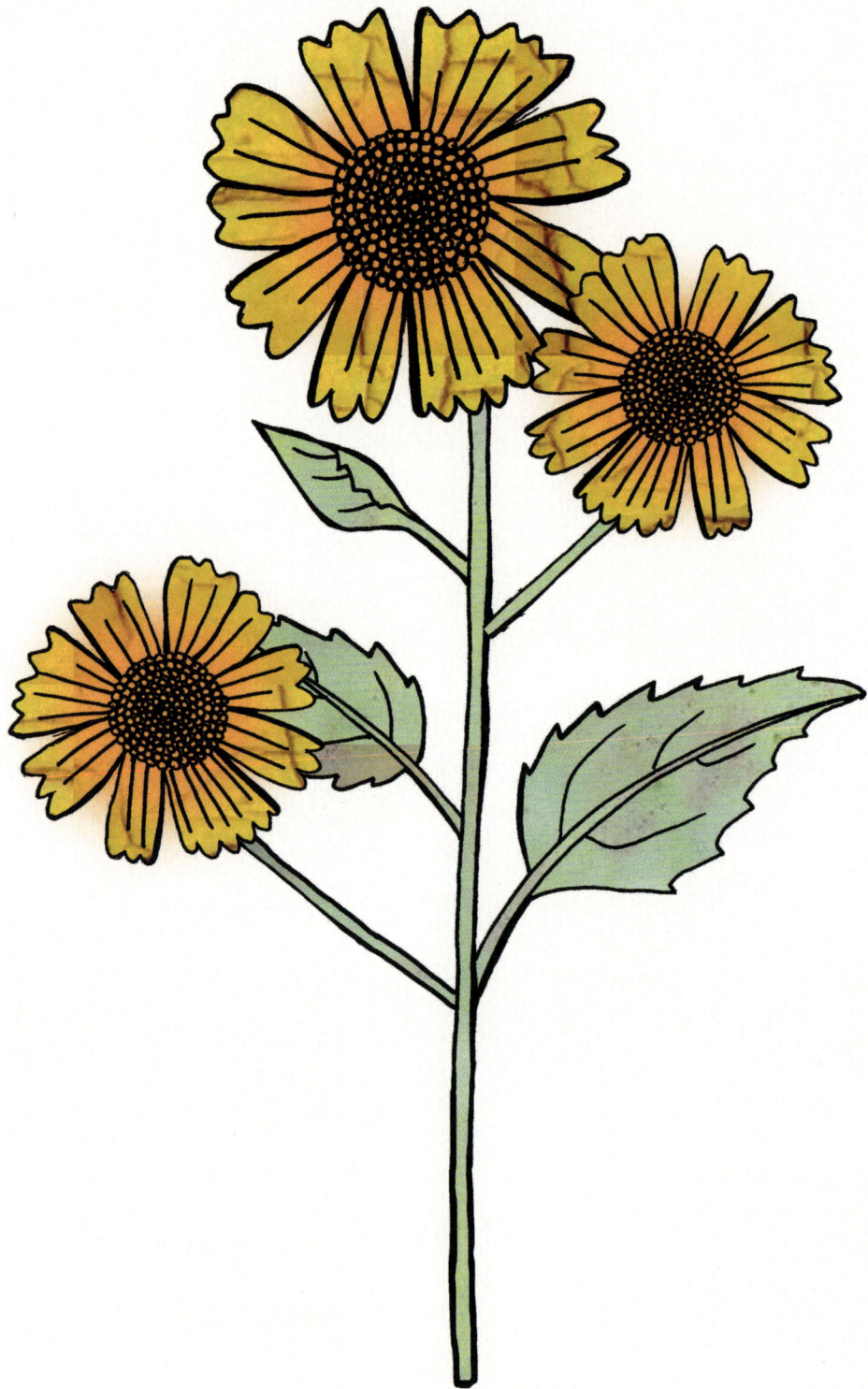

Cowpen Daisy

Verbesina encelioides

Appearance: This aster is a hardy, beautiful summer wildflower. They have silver-green leaves growing along a main stem that can grow up to 3 feet (91 cm) tall. They have bright-yellow flower heads with toothed petals in a circular formation around a disc. The flower heads can be up to 2 inches (5 cm) across and will continue to flower throughout the season. Their seeds are plentiful, which can lead to hundreds of daisies growing next to each other, putting on a spectacular show.

Habitat: Cowpen daisies have been found in thirty states throughout the United States and Mexico and tend to thrive in the Southwest. They grow in disturbed areas (like areas grazed by cows—thus their name) and sandy soils, usually found in lower elevations.

Blooming season: April through October.

Lifespan: It is considered an annual because the cold of winter will kill the plant, but it has a long lifespan, as it sprouts in early spring and dies off in late autumn.

Environmental roles: Cowpen daisies are great for desert restoration because they thrive in poor conditions that other wildflowers cannot and continually bloom for many months. They are an excellent source of nectar for pollinators, especially late-season butterflies like migrating monarchs, and are host plants for certain butterflies and moths. Cowpen daisies produce many seeds that native birds survive on.

Foraging: This plant was used externally by Indigenous peoples and early settlers to treat skin ailments (similar to other daisies). It can be mildly toxic if ingested. I love to spread seeds from this plant in my garden and yard because of how hardy it is.

Plant friends: Any plants in the aster family. Brittlebush is one example.

Creosote Bush

Larrea tridentata

Appearance: This well-known, sticky, green bush governs the Sonoran Desert. It can reach heights of up to 15 feet (4.5 m) and produces many tiny, pointed, waxy green leaves that produce an aromatic resin. This plant produces small, five-petal flowers after ample rainfall that can cover the bush.

Habitat: Sonoran, Chihuahuan, and Mojave Deserts in flat desert areas. Usually grows with many other creosote bushes under 5,000 feet (1,524 m) elevation.

Blooming season: Sporadically throughout the year.

Lifespan: Each bush can live up to ninety years, but since it reproduces through its roots as well as seeds, it can have clones of itself that are much, *much* older. There is a root system in the Mojave Desert that traces back 11,700 years, making the creosote bush one of the oldest living organisms on the planet.

Environmental roles: This plant is a desert necessity. Creosote bush helps prevent erosion, is the first long-living plant to establish itself in disturbed areas, and is a home and food base to over sixty species of insects and small wildlife. Their waxy leaves prevent water loss. Creosote bush flowers are the only food source for twenty-two species of bees because their flowers bloom throughout the year.

Foraging: Creosote bush is widely used by native and non-native desert dwellers. It has powerful medicinal properties. It is especially helpful for treating most kinds of skin issues, such as eczema, psoriasis, acne, small cuts, sunburns, bug bites, and even skin cancer (it is currently being studied for its anticarcinogenic properties). The aroma from the creosote bush has also been scientifically proven to reduce anxiety and help ground us.

Plant friends: Arizona poppy and other caltrop family members.

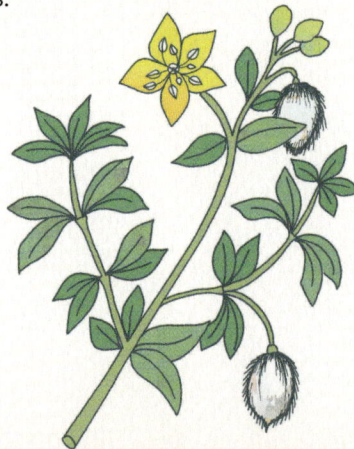

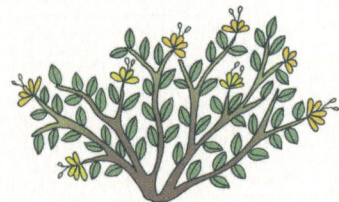

Creosote Bush Foraging, Oil, and Salve

Turn creosote bush into a healing oil or salve. To sustainably forage creosote bush, we must take only a small amount from each bush and only from healthy, green bushes. We can remove leaves and green stems (not the brown, thicker stems) to be used in extraction. I tend to take only from areas higher up on the bush to keep low coverage for wildlife. I follow the "no more than 10 percent of the plant" foraging rule, and most of the time I collect less.

MATERIALS

For the Oil

- Enough creosote bush leaves and green stems to fill half a jar

- Paper bag

- 1-quart (1 L) sterilized glass jar with lid

- 3 cups (720 ml) carrier oil (my favorite is jojoba oil)

- Fine-mesh strainer or tea cloth

For a Salve (Optional)

- ¾ cup (180 ml) creosote oil

- ½ ounce (15 g) beeswax

- Glass-pot double boiler

- Small jars or metal tins, for storage

INSTRUCTIONS

1. To make the oil: Rinse the foraged material, pat it dry, and place it in the paper bag. Let it sit until the actual plant material is crispy and dried. This could take 1 to 2 weeks depending on room temperature.

2. Fill the jar about halfway with the dried creosote bush.

3. Pour the carrier oil into the jar, completely covering the dried plant material. Screw the lid on tightly.

4. Place the jar in a dark space, such as a cupboard or paper bag, and let it extract for 1 month, or until the creosote bush is no longer bright green. The plant material will look very dark green, brown, or almost black. You can speed up the extraction process and possibly cut the extraction time in half by placing the jar (inside the paper bag) in the sun for heat (don't expose the jar to direct sunlight).

5. Once the oil extraction is ready, use a fine-mesh strainer or a tea cloth to strain the creosote out of the oil (the tea cloth will take longer).

6. Apply this creosote oil as is to heal skin issues.

7. To make a salve (optional): Add ¾ cup (60 ml) creosote oil and the beeswax to the pot of the glass-pot double boiler. Cook over medium-low heat, stirring often, until melted. Pour the melted mixture into small jars or metal tins and store.

Desert Senna

Senna covesii

Appearance: This adorable small shrub is covered in tiny gray hairs to help it retain moisture. It has a woody stalk with light grayish-green leaves, and its branches can grow up to 25 inches (63 cm) long. The yellow, veiny flowers surpass the size of the leaves, being about 1 inch (2.5 cm) across, and have five clawlike petals. Desert senna produces seeds in long, brownish pods that split open when dry to release the seeds.

Habitat: Found in Arizona, New Mexico, and California on dry rocky slopes, sandy desert washes, and mesas between 1,000 and 3,000 feet (305 and 914 m) elevation.

Blooming season: March through October.

Lifespan: Perennial that can live for a few years.

Environmental roles: Desert senna is a great source of nectar for pollinators and insects because of its long, continual blooming cycle. Its seeds are also a source of food for desert rodents and birds.

Foraging: Senna plants can be used medicinally in teas or tinctures as a stimulant and laxative. Desert senna is considered rare or endangered in California because of vehicles and road maintenance. Though not endangered in Arizona, please keep foraging to a minimum.

Plant friends: Twinleaf senna and woolly senna.

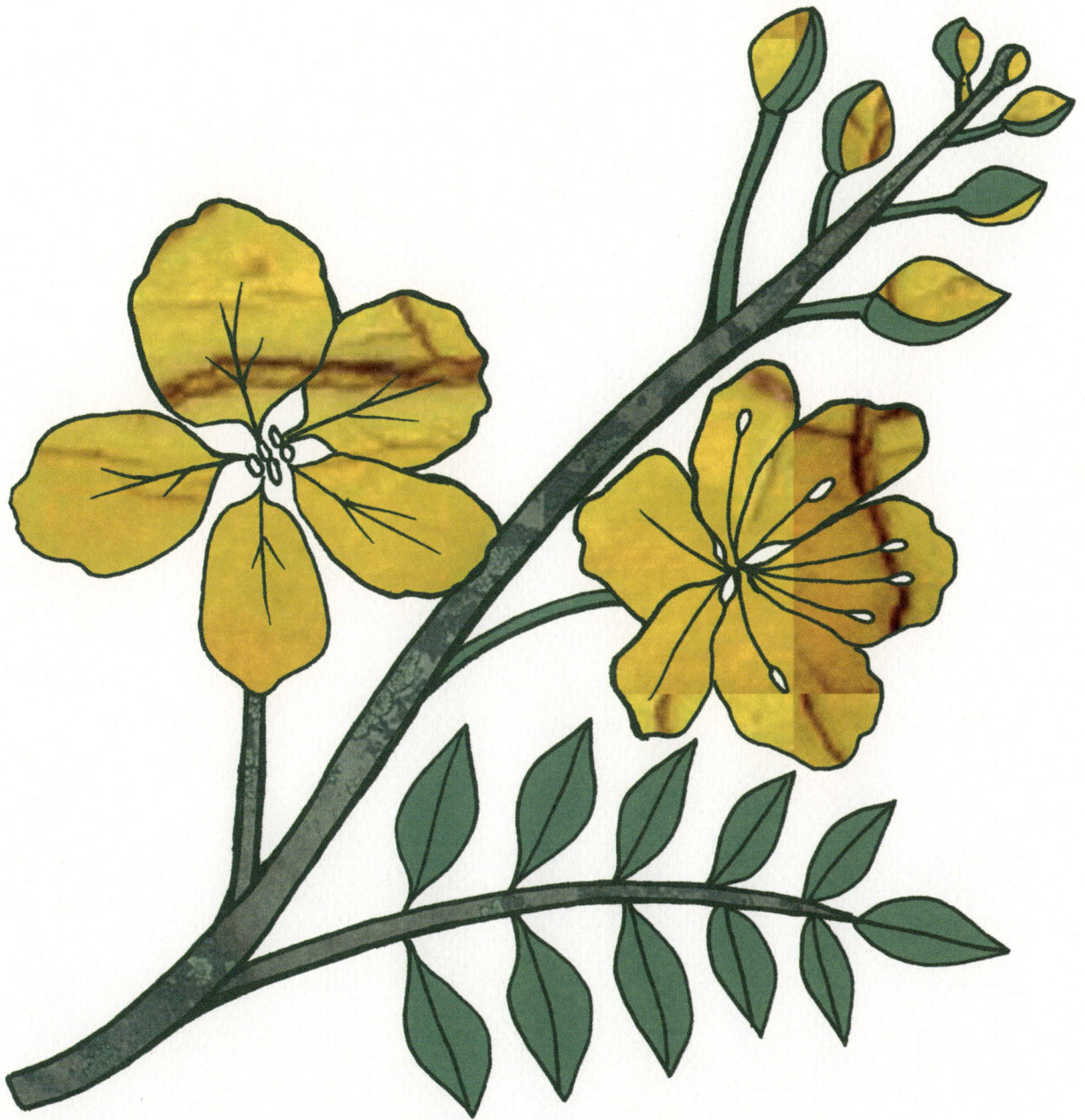

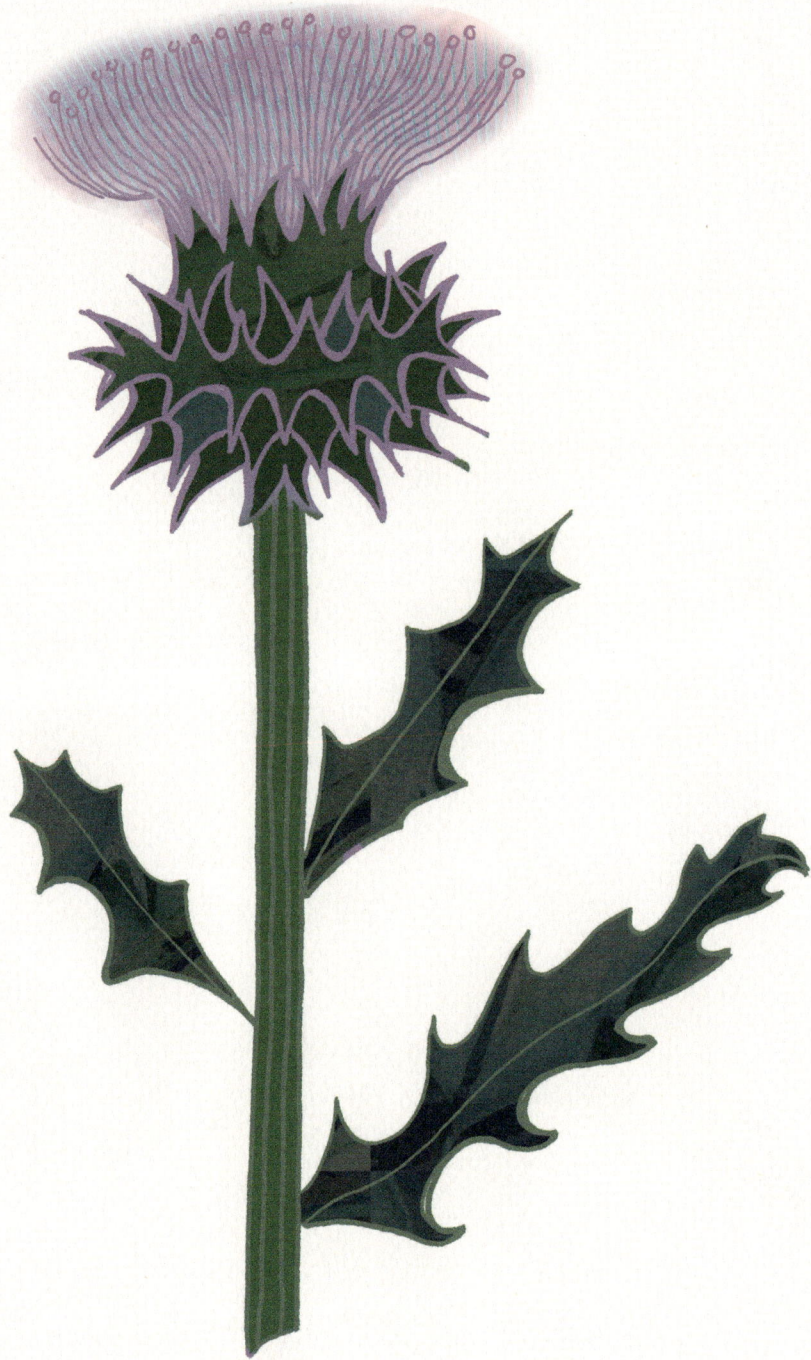

Desert Thistle or New Mexico Thistle

Cirsium neomexicanum

Appearance: These spiny plants are unique. Desert thistle has a long main stem covered in long, stiff, sharp spines with oblong, greenish-gray leaves that are also covered in spines. They can grow up to 6 feet (1.8 m) tall. The showy bright-fuchsia flower heads are about 2 to 3 inches (5 to 7.5 cm) wide and are surrounded by sharp spines. They grow solitary or with two to three other flower heads. The flowers have thin, fluffy-looking petals, bunched together, like other thistles.

Habitat: Found throughout the Sonoran, Chihuahuan, and Mojave Deserts. Residing in many different habitats like plains, hillsides, washes, and urban areas between 1,000 and 6,500 feet (305 and 1,981 m).

Blooming season: March through September.

Lifespan: Less than two years.

Environmental roles: Desert thistle and other thistles support a variety of native pollinators (including bats). Its longer life cycle provides food from its leaves, seeds, and stems for insects. Songbirds feed off the seeds and also make nests from the thistle's down (fluffy material produced by the flower head).

Foraging: Thistles are related to artichokes and are most definitely edible. The young stalks and taproots are healthy sources of food for us humans. The harvesting window is short, as the taproots are best foraged in young plants and can be dug up and eaten raw or cooked. The root is known to the Navajo as "life medicine." The stalks are best when the plant is only about 1 to 2 feet (30.5 to 61 cm) tall because waiting longer means the stalks will be too fibrous. This plant is spiky, so it is important to wear gloves while collecting and de-thorn the stalks before eating. Stalks can be peeled and eaten fresh or cooked like asparagus and have a crisp, nutty flavor.

Plant friends: Arizona thistle and Graham's thistle.

Desert Willow

Chilopsis linearis

Appearance: This gorgeous desert tree can grow up to 40 feet (12 m) tall with a twisting trunk, slender branches, and a spreading canopy. The light green leaves are long and slender and can grow up to 1 foot (30.5 cm) long and about ⅓ inch (8 mm) wide. They have no thorns, unlike so many other desert trees. The flowers are funnel shaped and about 1½ inches (4 cm) long, and ruffled with petallike lobes. They range in color from light purple to dark pink with white or yellow streaks and have a lovely, violet-like scent. The flowers turn into slender seedpods in the autumn, about 6 to 10 inches (15 to 25 cm) long.

Habitat: Found in the Sonoran and Chihuahuan Deserts in ditches, arroyos, swales, washes, and desert areas, up to 5,000 feet (1,524 m).

Blooming season: April through October (peak blooming between May and June).

Lifespan: Ranges from 20 to 150 years.

Environmental roles: This fast-growing tree is used throughout desert city landscaping because it can thrive in a variety of soil conditions with very minimal water and can prevent soil erosion. Its flowers provide rich nectar for pollinators like hummingbirds. It produces seeds for other native birds as well.

Foraging: This tree has many uses. Indigenous peoples use the wood from the desert willow to create bows and baskets. A tea made from its flowers can soothe coughs. Its leaves and stems can be used in salves or washes for wounds because of its antifungal, antimicrobial properties. Tinctures can be made to help treat candida and valley fever.

Plant friends: Yellowbells, trumpet creeper.

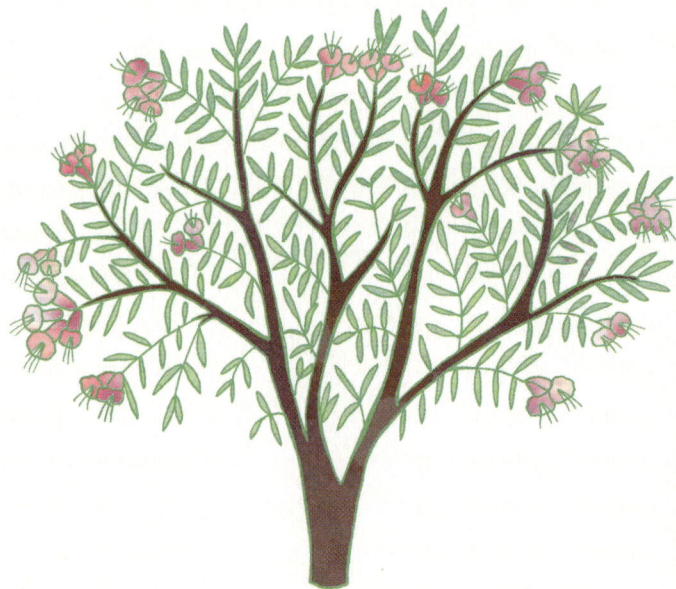

Willow Facial Toner

This toner can help keep your skin clear and reduce redness as it gets rid of bad bacteria and supports healthy probiotics.

MATERIALS

- Desert willow tree leaves and flowers (or just leaves, depending on season); enough to fill the jar halfway

- 16-ounce (0.5 L) sterilized jar with lid

- 1¼ cups (300 ml) apple cider vinegar

- Strainer

- Essential oil(s), such as lavender or orange (optional)

INSTRUCTIONS

1. Rinse the foraged leaves and flowers and add them to the jar, filling the jar about halfway.

2. Pour the apple cider vinegar into the jar, covering the leaves completely. Screw the jar lid on tightly, then let it sit and extract in a dark place for at least 2 weeks.

3. Once the decoction is done, strain the leaves out with the strainer.

4. Use as is or add 5 to 8 drops of essential oil(s).

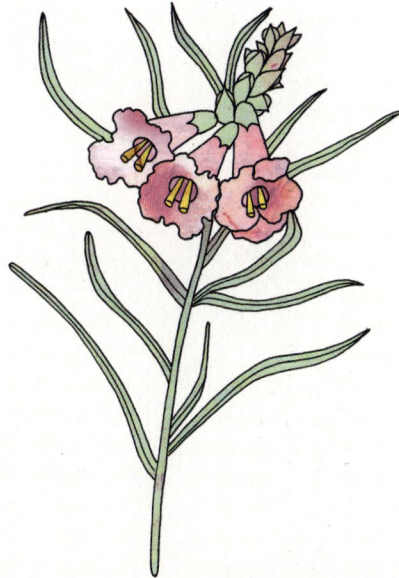

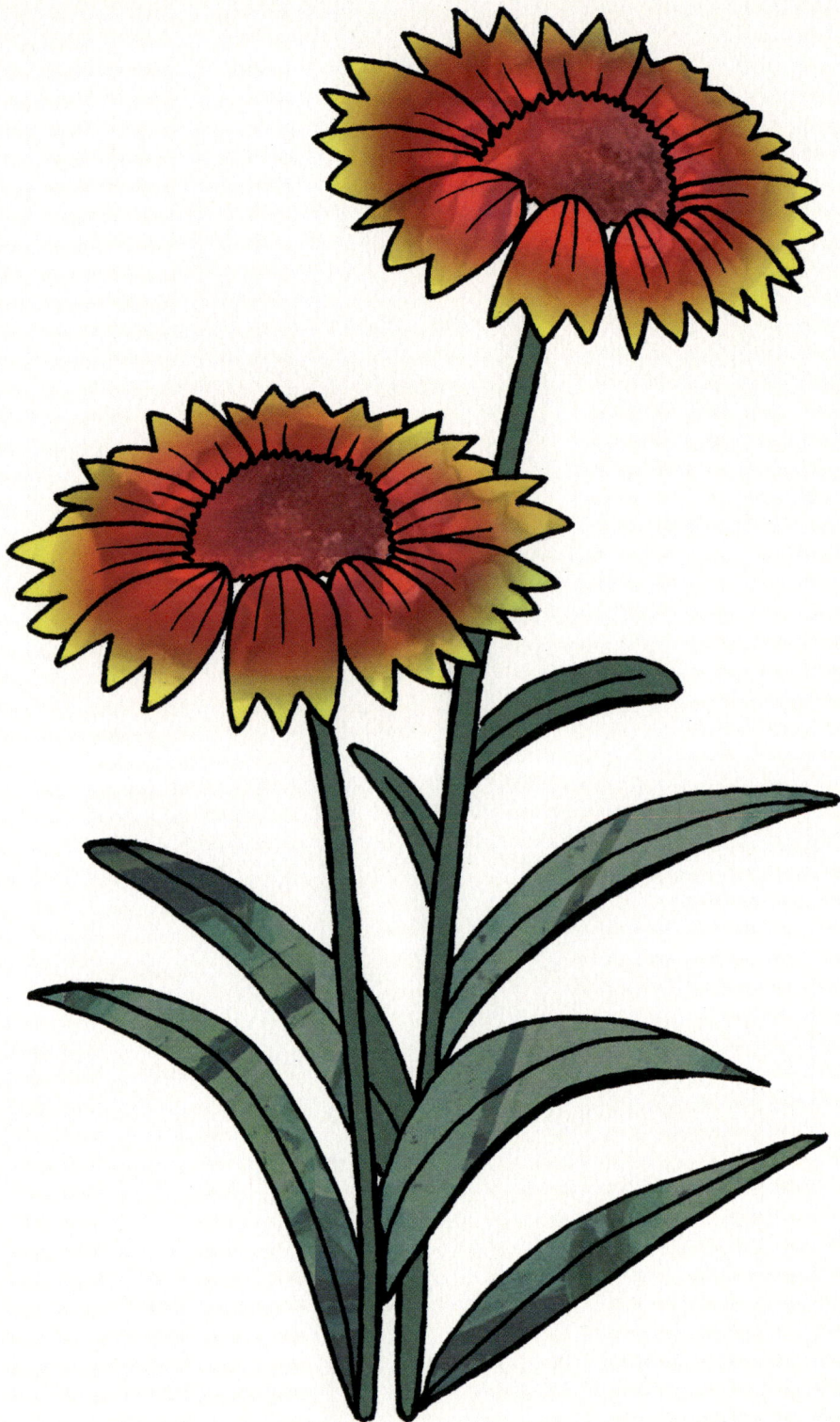

Firewheel

Gaillardia pulchella

Appearance: These bright pinwheel flowers stand 1 to 2 feet (30.5 to 61 cm) tall, with a hairy branched stem with green leaves. They have fiery flower heads with rays (petals) that are red at the base and yellow at the toothed tips that surround a brownish-red disc. Firewheels are most definitely an exciting find!

Habitat: They are widespread, distributed throughout much of the United States and Mexico in dry plains and open areas in well-draining soil between 3,500 and 5,500 feet (1,067 to 1,676 m) elevation.

Blooming season: April through August.

Lifespan: Mostly an annual, though some can live a couple of years.

Environmental roles: Firewheel is drought tolerant and known for growing in poor conditions, so it makes for a great restoration plant. It also hosts pollinators like butterflies and moths. Its seeds are a food source for birds and small mammals.

Foraging: Firewheel root is beneficial for skin disorders and the stems and flowers can be used as anti-inflammatories. They aren't super common in Arizona, as they tend to grow at higher elevations in and surrounding the sky islands, so forage to a minimum.

Plant friends: Red dome blanketflower.

Graham's Nipple Cactus

Mammillaria grahamii

Appearance: These inconspicuous, tiny, greenish-gray cacti grow in tubular barrel shapes less than 1 foot (30.5 cm) tall, with purplish hooked spines that cover the whole body. They usually grow in clusters. They wear a flower crown of bright-pink fringed flowers, usually no more than 1 inch (2.5 cm) across, after adequate monsoon rainfall. The flowers do not stick around for long and quickly turn into elongated red fruits that almost resemble small chilis, but taste slightly sweet and have the texture of a strawberry.

Habitat: Sonoran Desert in a variety of habitats, but mostly in grasslands or rocky, sandy, or gravelly slopes here in southern Arizona between 3,000 and 4,500 feet (91 to 1,372 m) elevation. Typically found growing under and with the creosote bush.

Blooming season: April through September, but tend to bloom in late July here in Tucson.

Lifespan: Unknown, though likely at least five years or more.

Environmental roles: This Mammillaria is a tough little plant and easy to propagate, making it perfect for desert landscaping. Its fruits are food for small mammals and birds like the greater roadrunner.

Foraging: The fruits of Graham's nipple cactus are edible and have been eaten by Indigenous peoples for thousands of years. I forage the occasional fruit in autumn when they are ripe, but tend to leave most for wildlife. They are a tasty, tiny treat with a slightly sweet and bitter taste.

Plant friends: Thornber's nipple cactus.

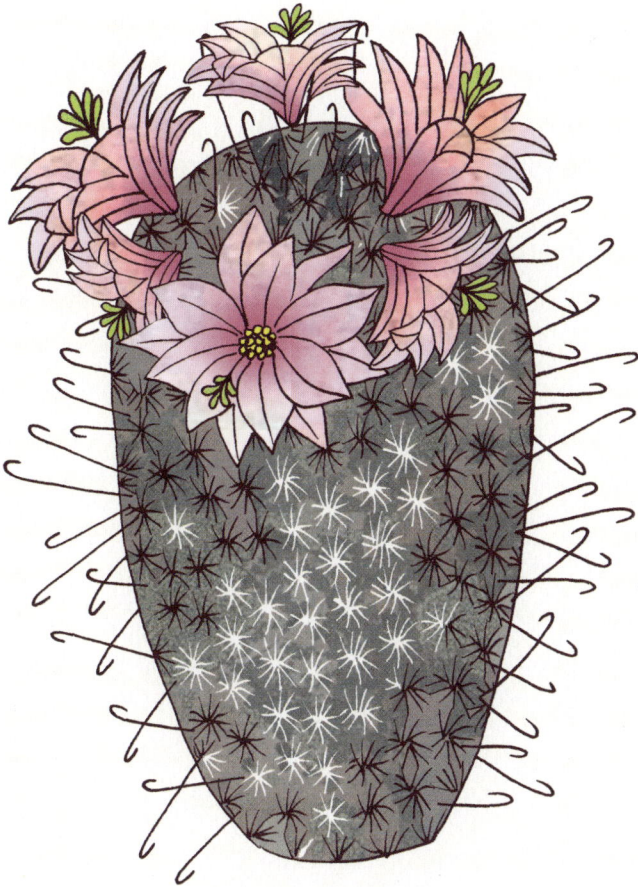

Graham's Nipple Cactus

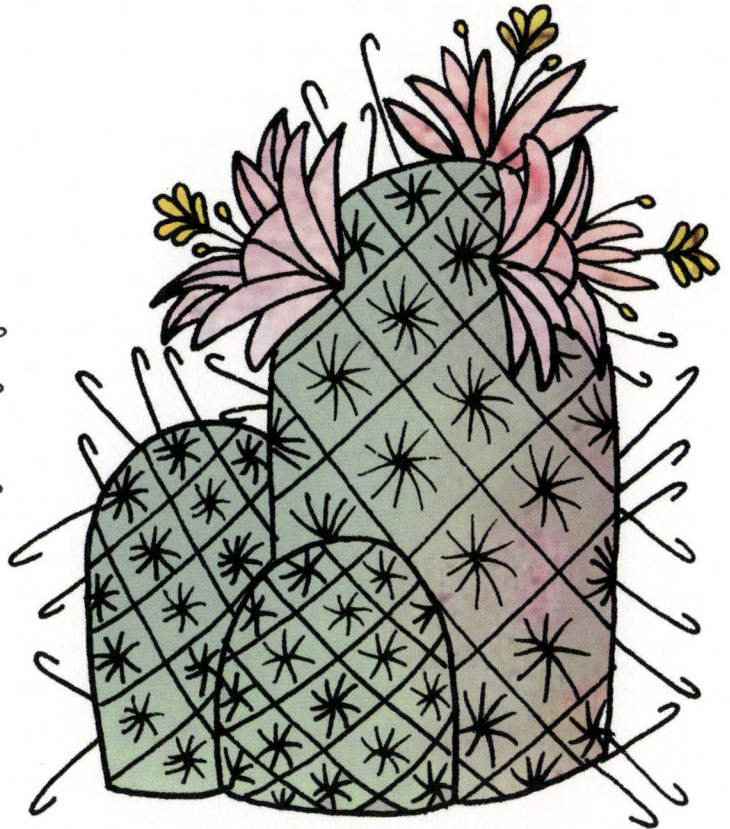

Rarer Thornber's Nipple Cactus

Difference Between Graham's Nipple Cactus and the Rarer Thornber's Nipple Cactus

Thornber's nipple cactus looks similar to Graham's nipple cactus but is smaller, growing only about 4 inches (10 cm) tall in dense clumps. Its flowers are also smaller and a lighter pink color. Thornber's can only be found in a small area in the Saguaro National Park West and on the Tohono O'odham reservation in Arizona, and is therefore considered endangered.

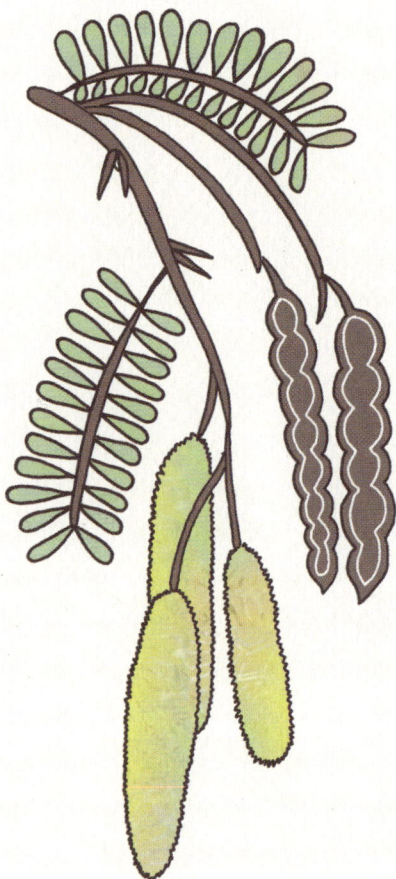

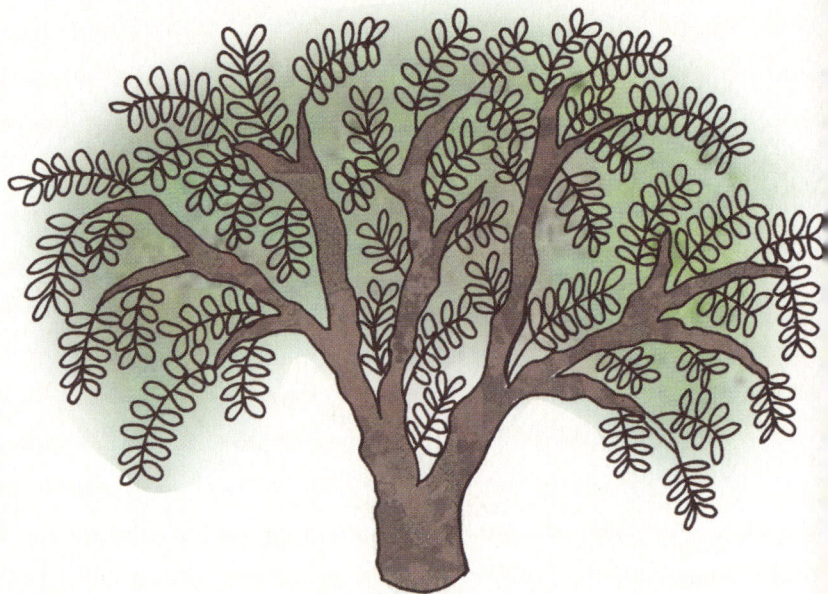

Mesquite Flour

A delicious and healthy flour comes from mesquite beans (or seed pods). The beans are harvested once they are dried and still hanging on the tree. They need to be fully dried before they are then ground using a mill into a flour, and the hard seeds and leftover shells are removed with a sifter. Mesquite flour can be used in baking on its own but tastes a lot better when mixed with other flours because it has a strong taste. I like to add mesquite flour to pancakes, banana bread, and cookies.

Velvet Mesquite Tree

Neltuma velutina

Appearance: Velvet mesquites are the Sonoran Desert's tallest growing and most common mesquite, growing up to 50 feet (15 m) tall. This tree grows a large spreading crown with zigzagged branches that are covered in pairs of spines. The bark is a reddish-brown color with a shaggy, thick, rough texture. The small green leaflets grow off thin stems in a feather-like pattern. It blooms long, pale-yellow, fluffy, puff-like flowers that release a lot of pollen which is then carried by the wind (causing allergies in some humans). They produce edible, slender, curved seed pods that are beige in color with purplish streaks along the edges.

Habitat: Sonoran, Mojave, and Chihuahuan Deserts, but can be found more densely in southern Arizona in desert washes, grasslands, riparian areas, and canyons in sandy or rocky soil, mostly below 4,500 feet (1,372 m).

Blooming season: April through June.

Lifespan: Can live up to two hundred years!

Environmental roles: Velvet mesquites are essential for our desert environment. They tend to grow together with many other velvet mesquites in what are called "bosques," which provide shade and shelter to tons of desert plants and dwellers (it can be ten degrees cooler under a tree). They produce a lot of edible, sweet, protein-rich seed pods which help feed wildlife like coyotes and other small mammals, and have fed Indigenous peoples for thousands of years. They are partly pollinated by bees that produce delicious honey when they thrive on mostly mesquite flowers. The tree's hardwood is great for building all kinds of decorations, furniture, and structures.

Foraging: Velvet mesquites are widely harvested for their edible seed pods, which can be ground into flour and added to a variety of meals and baked goods. The flour has a slightly sweet, earthy taste. The hardwood from fallen trees can be harvested to create long-lasting mesquite furniture, decoration, or other home goods, and also makes great charcoal that, when burned, flavors food with its smoke.

Plant friends: Screwbean mesquite and honey mesquite.

Mt. Lemmon Marigold

Tagetes lemmonii

Appearance: Mt. Lemmon marigold is endemic to a small area of the Sonoran Desert. It is a bushy evergreen shrub that can grow up to 6 feet (1.8 m) tall. It has very fragrant foliage that has a bright, citrusy, camphor scent. It has soft, thin, vibrant green leaves and eight-petal, daisylike, dark-yellow flowers.

Habitat: Southern Arizona and northern Mexico in the sky islands at about 4,000 to 8,000 feet (1,219 to 2,438 m) elevation.

Blooming season: June through September

Lifespan: Can live up to five years.

Environmental roles: Mt. Lemmon marigold is a food source for pollinators, birds, and beneficial insects. Its strong scent deters rabbits and deer.

Foraging: Practitioners of herbal medicine use this plant in a tea to soothe stomach pains and inflammation. Its flowers can be used in salves to help heal bruises, minor skin injuries, and inflammation. I would use this plant very sparingly, as it is not very common, unless cultivated in a home garden or desert nursery.

Plant friends: All marigolds (tagetes).

Sky islands of the Sonoran Desert

Sky islands are desert mountains at higher elevations. They are surrounded by desert or grasslands, but their biomes are very different as elevation increases. They are unique to the Sonoran Desert. Sky islands are a wealth of biodiversity and the Coronado National Forest, which includes most of the sky islands, is the most ecologically diverse national forest in the United States. The flora and fauna that live in the sky islands could not survive the climate below it. I personally love driving up sky islands like Mt. Graham and Mt. Lemmon to witness the biomes change from desert, to chaparral, to temperate deciduous forest, to coniferous forest, all within an hour's drive. The temperature change is dramatic, as well, with temperatures dropping up to thirty degrees at the highest altitudes. These unique oases are favorite places for desert dwellers to escape to in the heat of the summer.

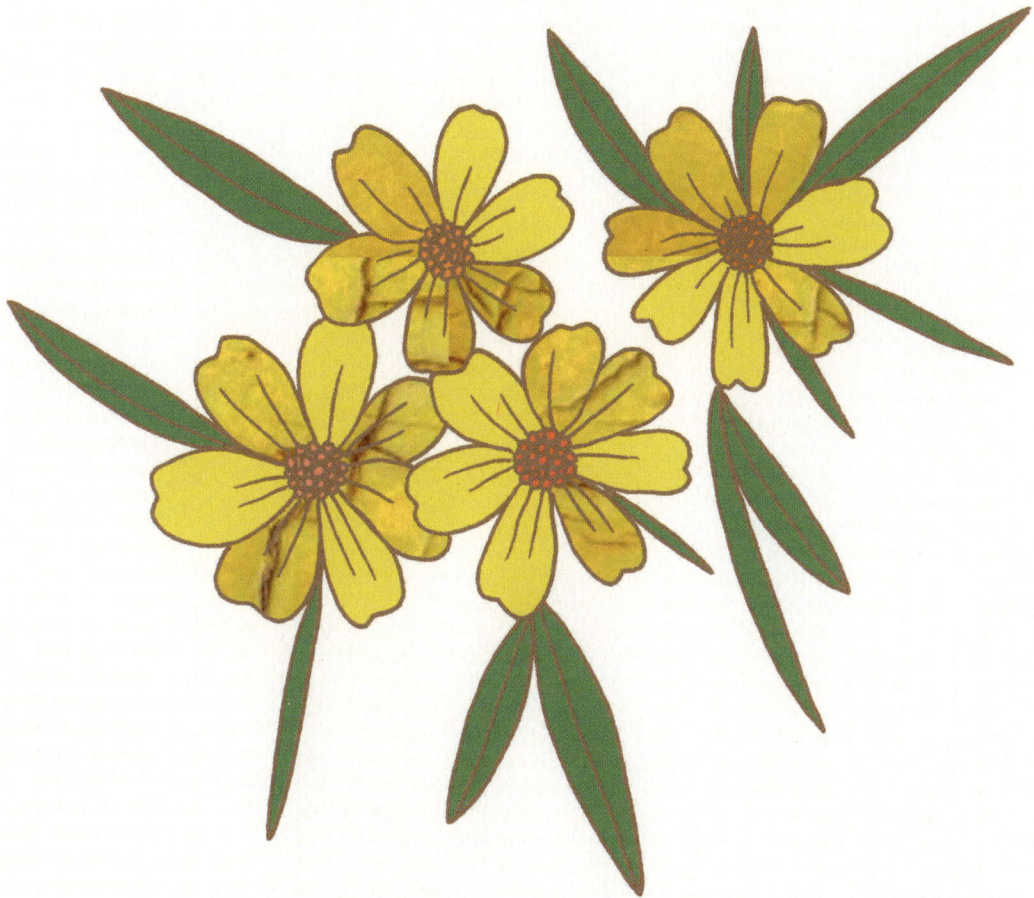

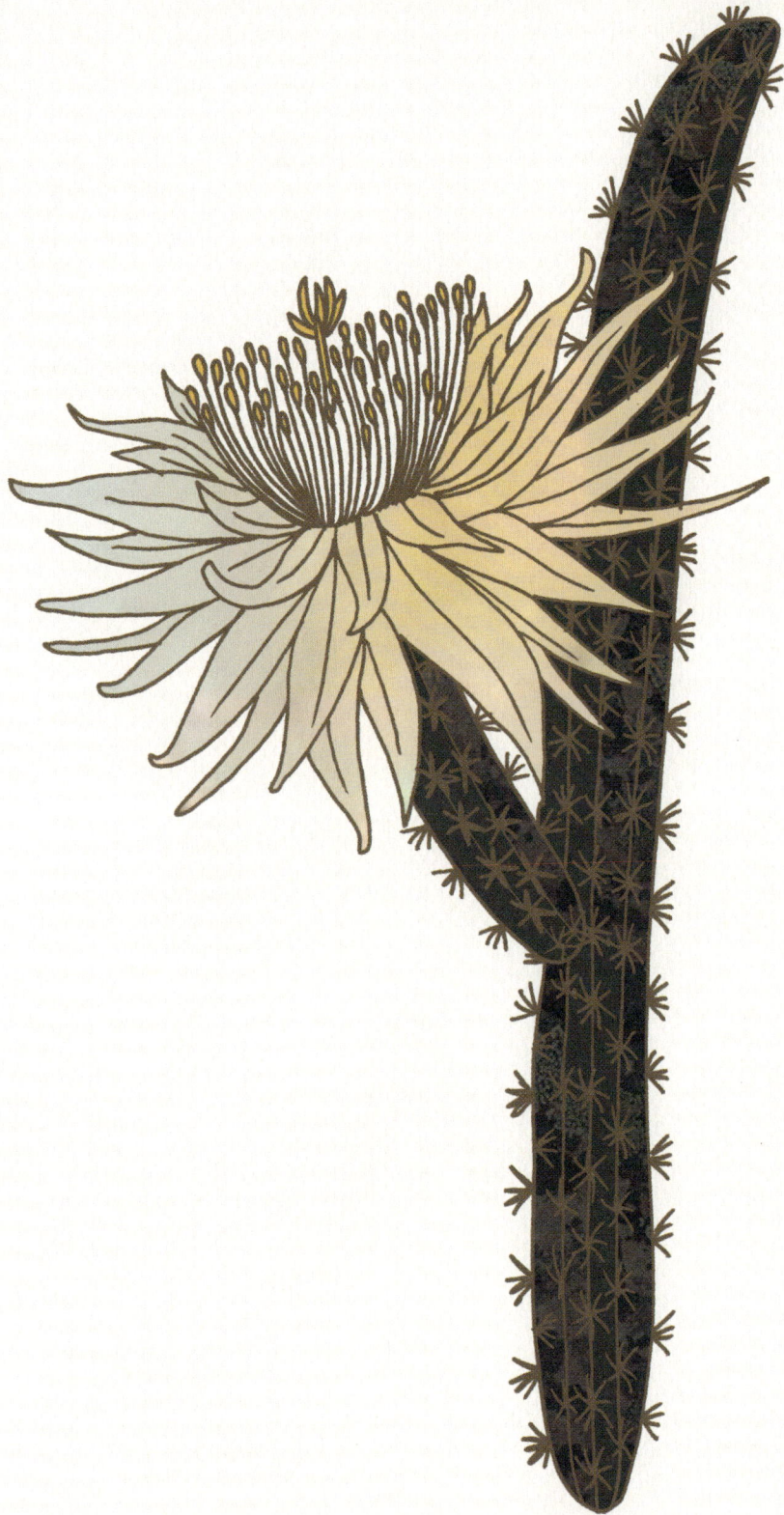

Night-Blooming Cereus

Peniocereus greggii

Appearance: This rare cactus only has a few long, slender, purplish-gray stems that are armed with short, dark spines along its four to six ribs. It can grow up to 3 feet (91 cm) tall. These cacti can go unnoticed from its surrounding habitat except when they bloom a few spectacular giant white flowers about 3 inches (7.5 cm) across, which only open for one night. The flowers have a strong vanilla scent. The night-blooming cereus is widely sought after, to witness its blooms.

Habitat: Primarily found in the Sonoran Desert growing with creosote bush at elevations below 4,000 feet (1,219 m).

Blooming season: Late June to early July.

Lifespan: Can live up to a few years.

Environmental roles: The fruit of the night-blooming cereus is consumed by native wildlife. The large flowers and strong scent attract hawk moths for pollination.

Foraging: This plant is considered threatened in native habitats because of urban development, pollinator scarcity, and collectors digging up entire plants. Please do not forage.

Plant friends: Arizona queen of the night cactus.

Engelmann Prickly Pear Cactus

Opuntia engelmanii

Appearance: These iconic bushy succulents have bluish-green, egg-shaped, fleshy pads up to 1 foot (30.5 cm) across. The pads are covered in white clusters of spines about 1 inch (2.5 cm) long, with glochids covering the base of the clusters. In spring, they grow masses of stunning yellow flowers up to 2 inches (5 cm) in diameter along the edges of the pads. The flowers then turn into edible, juicy, purplish-red fruits up to 2 inches (5 cm) long. The fruits (tunas) are often harvested from this cactus and are a desert delicacy.

Habitat: Southern United States and northern Mexico in sandy, gravelly soils at about 1,000 to 9,000 feet (305 to 2,743 m) elevation.

Blooming season: Flowers April through June, and fruit July through September.

Lifespan: Can live up to fifty-five years.

Environmental roles: These prickly pears offer hydrating, vitamin-rich fruits. These cacti retain moisture very easily and are extremely drought tolerant. They can propagate themselves just from a pad falling on the ground. The flowers offer pollen for native bees as well as protection for packrats as they dig their burrows under and through the root system.

Foraging: Native people of the Sonoran Desert use these fruits as a food source. Foraging these fruits in a sustainable way is very important. The fruits become ripe usually in August (they are dark purple and the juice is magenta when the fruit is squeezed). I use tongs to collect them and only take a few from the tops of each cactus, leaving low-hanging fruit for wildlife. I try to find large patches of prickly pears so I can forage enough fruit to juice.

Plant friends: Santa Rita prickly pear cactus.

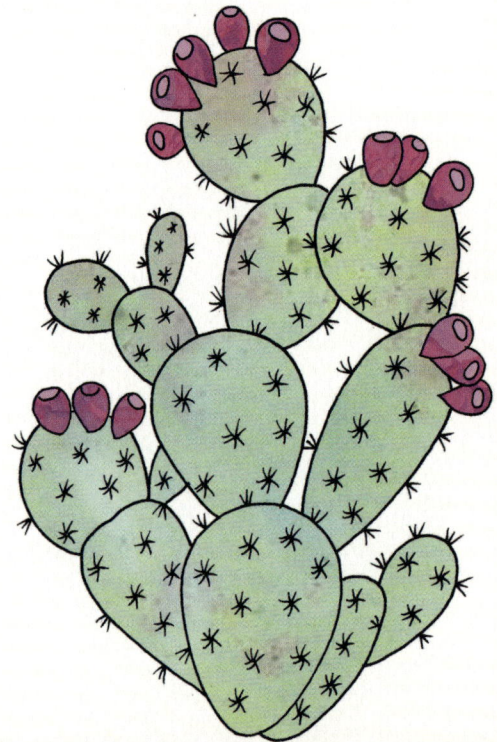

Easy Prickly Pear Fruit Juice

Prickly pear juice is high in electrolytes and vitamins, which makes it great for late summer, after we have been experiencing high temperatures for months. It is a perfect example of the desert providing exactly what we need at the right time.

MATERIALS

- About 1 gallon-size (3.8 L) bag prickly pears
- Airtight freezable container or resealable plastic bag
- 2 large bowls, divided
- Paring knife
- Potato masher or pestle
- Tongs
- Colander
- Very fine-mesh strainer or tea strainer
- Sterilized glass jar with lid (large enough for strained juice)
- 2 tablespoons lime juice or 1 teaspoon citric acid (optional)

INSTRUCTIONS

1. Rinse the prickly pears well, place them inside the airtight container and freeze for at least 2 weeks.

2. After 2 weeks, thaw the prickly pears and dump them into one of the large bowls. Use the paring knife to gently slice each pear open down the middle (be careful of pressure and juice squirting everywhere).

3. Use the potato masher or pestle to smash the pears well.

4. Place the colander inside the other large bowl. Use the tongs to place smashed pears in the colander to strain the juice. You can use the potato masher to press the remaining juice from the skin and seeds. When finished, compost or throw the skins and seeds into a yard for wildlife to find.

5. Strain the juice again through the fine-mesh strainer (as fine as a tea strainer) into the jar; this removes the tiny glochids.

6. You now have pure prickly pear juice! Use within 2 weeks; you can add some lime juice or citric acid to get the juice to last longer in the fridge, or you can freeze whatever you aren't currently using. (I also sell Prickly Pear Fruit Concentrate year-round, if you want to save yourself all this hassle).

Desert Horsepurslane
Trianthema portulacastrum

Appearance: Desert horsepurslane is a semi succulent herb that grows in a mat formation, low to the ground, no higher than 18 inches (46 cm) tall. The stems are a waxy magenta color and its green leaves are oval shaped or round. The purple flowers are tiny and trumpet shaped. Fruits are capsules that burst to spread the seeds when dry enough.

Habitat: Most of the United States and Mexico in moist areas after heavy rainfall, between 1,000 and 4,000 feet (305 and 1,219 m).

Blooming season: June through October.

Lifespan: Annual.

Environmental roles: This plant is fast-growing in summertime but also doesn't live long. It makes a great source of food for wildlife and humans. It is sometimes considered a noxious "weed," but I don't believe any native plant to be a weed because they all play an important role in the ecosystem.

Foraging: The young leaves of this plant can be eaten raw or cooked. I like to add them to salads or cook them with eggs. This plant contains more vitamins than spinach. The roots have been used to treat stomach and liver ailments and asthma. The leaves can be used to treat anemia (probably because it is rich in iron), throat pain, fungal infections, and more. This plant is a lifesaver in the summer and not bad tasting, although the non-native common purslane does have a slightly better taste to it. Forage freely.

Plant friends: Common purslane.

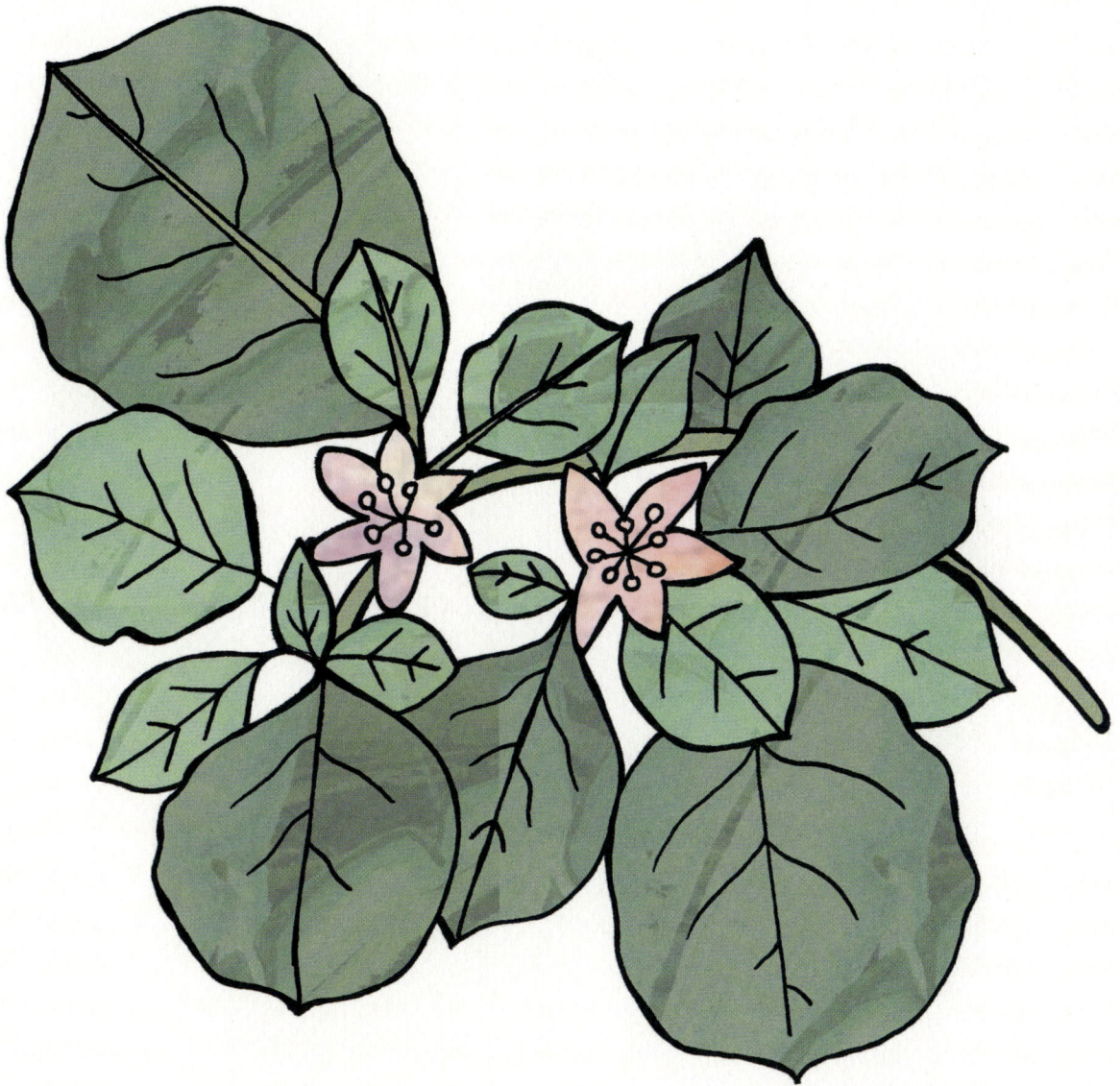

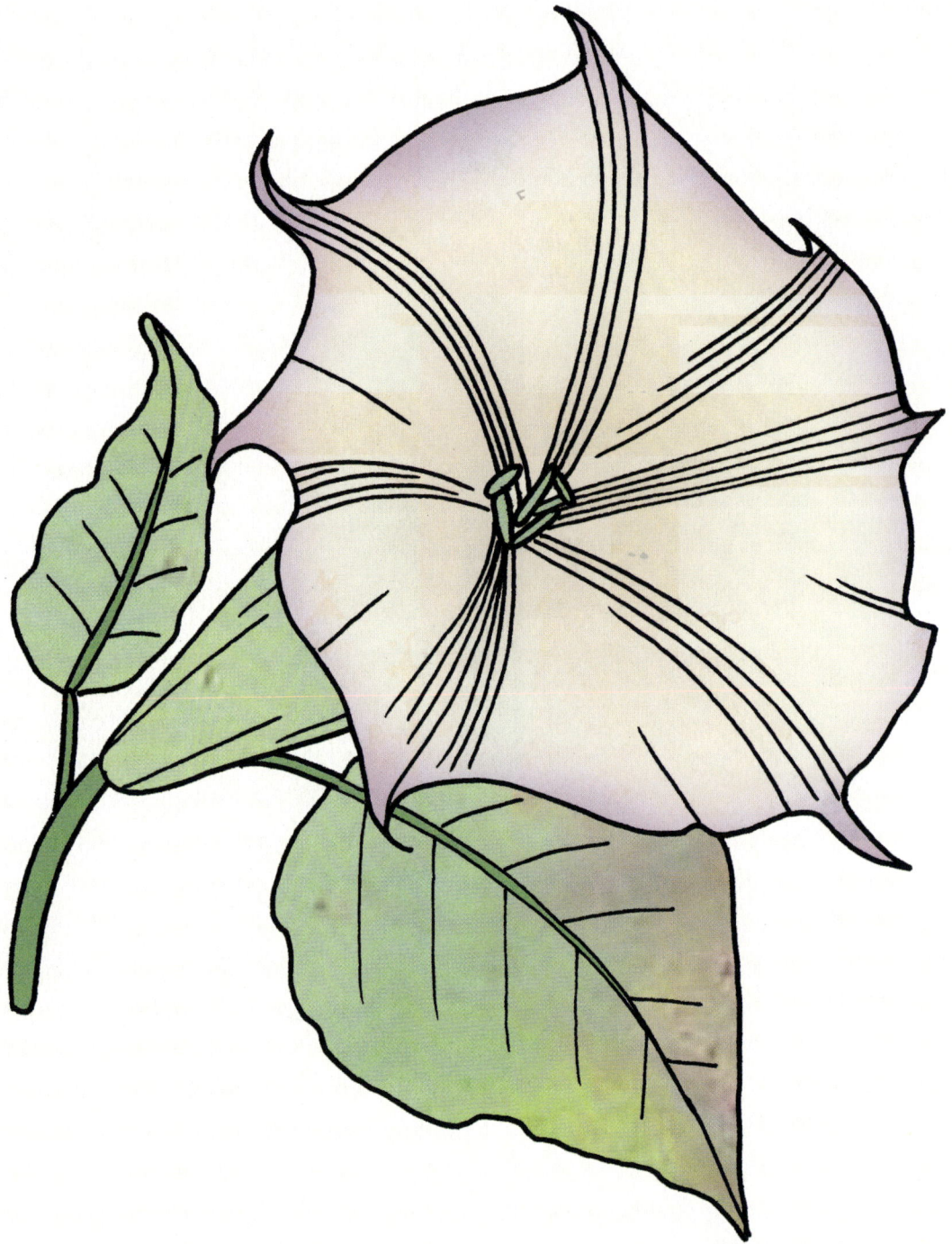

Sacred Datura

Datura wrightii

Appearance: This sprawling, night-blooming beauty is known for its magic. The entire plant can grow up to 6 feet (1.8 m) tall and 10 feet (3 m) wide. The triangular leaves are green but have a gray sheen because of the tiny white hairs and are less than 4.5 inches (11 cm) long. Sacred datura is most well known for its large, fragrant trumpet flowers, which grow up to 8 inches (20 cm) long and are white with faint lavender edges. Petals are fused together and form five sharp points symmetrically arranged around the margin. Once the blooming season is over, the flowers turn into green, ball-shaped seed pods about 1½ inches (4 cm) across that are covered with long, hooked spines. Once the seed pod dries, it splits open to release the seeds.

Habitat: Southwestern United States and northern Mexico in well-draining soil between 1,000 and 6,000 feet (305 to 1,829 m).

Blooming season: April through October.

Lifespan: Can live a few years but are mostly considered annuals, as they die off with the cold and reemerge from seed in the spring.

Environmental roles: This plant is an important nectar source to hawk moths, as it is one of the few desert night-bloomers.

Foraging: A true moonflower, this plant is considered toxic to humans, darkly hallucinogenic, and could cause death. Do not forage.

Plant friends: Any nightshades (the Solanaceae family).

Saguaro Fruit

Carnegiea gigantea / Bahidaj (Tohono O'odham name)

Appearance: The tallest beings in the desert will be crowned on almost every arm with fruit during the hottest months of the summer. (See page 50 for a detailed description of Saguaro cacti.) The fruits are green to red on the outside and are oval-shaped, with a dried flower on top. They are about 2 to 3½ inches (5 to 9 cm) long and 1 to 2 inches (2.5 to 5 cm) wide. When they ripen and split open, they are filled with a bright-red, juicy pulp, filled with up to two thousand small seeds that resemble poppy seeds.

Habitat: Exclusively in the Sonoran Desert, mostly in southern Arizona and western Sonora, Mexico. They live between sea level and 4,500 feet (1,372 m) elevation.

Ripening season: Mid-June to early July.

Lifespan: The fruits are only available in specific parts of June and July.

Environmental roles: The Tohono O'odham have survived off saguaro fruit every summer for thousands of years and deeply revere these cacti for all they provide. The saguaro fruits are also essential for desert wildlife to survive the harsh summer months. They provide food for birds, bats, coyotes, javelinas, tortoises, and insects like millipedes. They are filled with electrolytes, which provide essential moisture before the monsoon rains later in the summer. The saguaro is a keystone species, so the spreading of the seeds from the fruit are vital to the Sonoran ecosystem.

Foraging: Foraging saguaro fruit in minimal amounts is acceptable. The Saguaro National Park allows visitors to harvest small amounts for immediate consumption. I tend to get permission from private property owners if I want to taste a few. As described above, these fruits are vital to the ecosystem, so taking more than a few is frowned upon. A long pole, stick, or saguaro rib is needed to knock a ripe fruit off a low-hanging saguaro arm. A technique I learned from a Pascua Yaqui friend is to remove the dried saguaro flower from the fruit and use the disclike end to slice open the fruit. The entire inside pulp can be eaten, seeds and all. They are thirst-quenching, tasty treats on a hot summer day, and the ripest ones can be very sweet.

Plant friends: Saguaros are the only plant in the Carnegiea genus but are related to all other cacti in the Cactaceae family, like the barrel cactus and the cardon cactus.

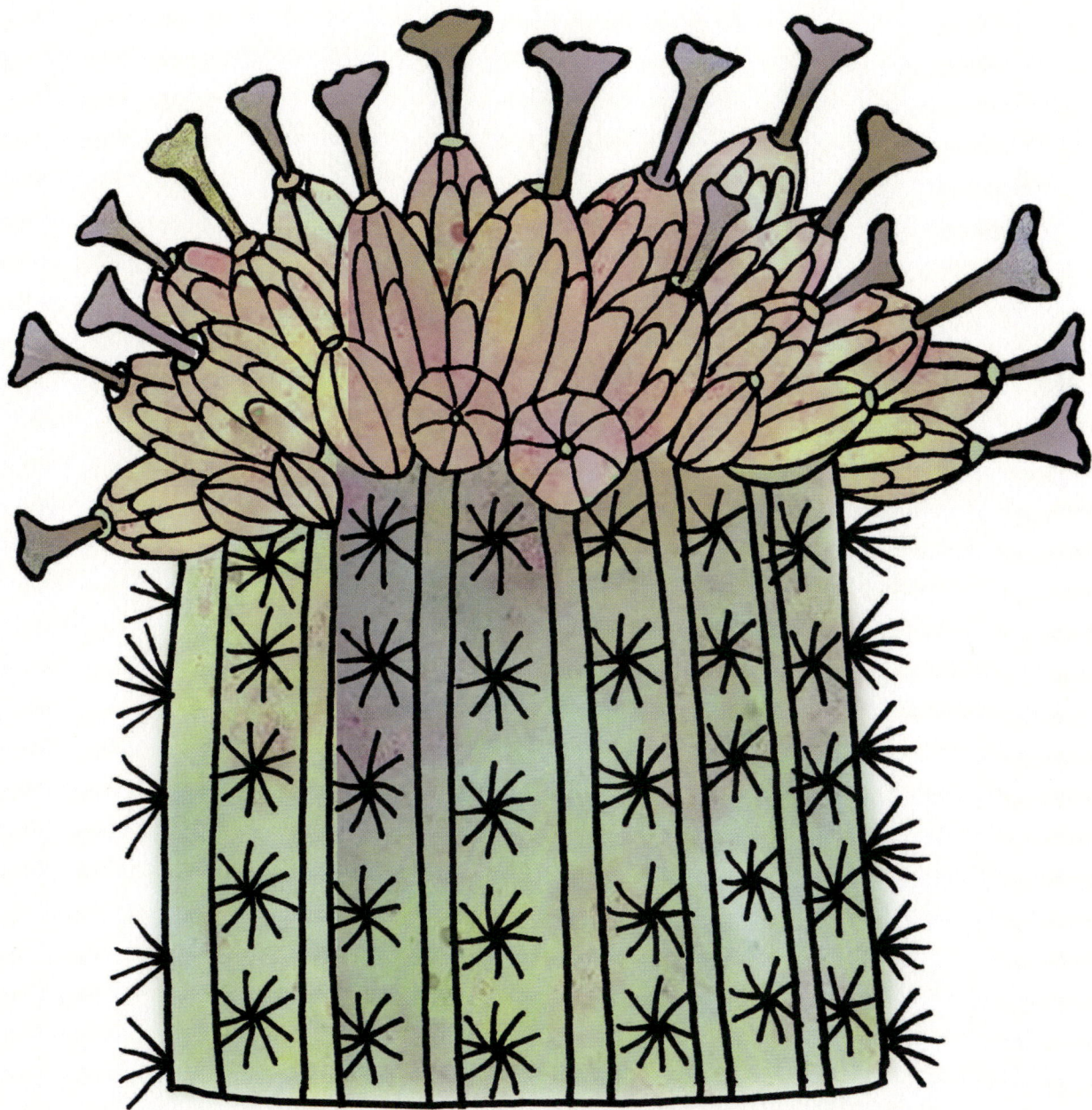

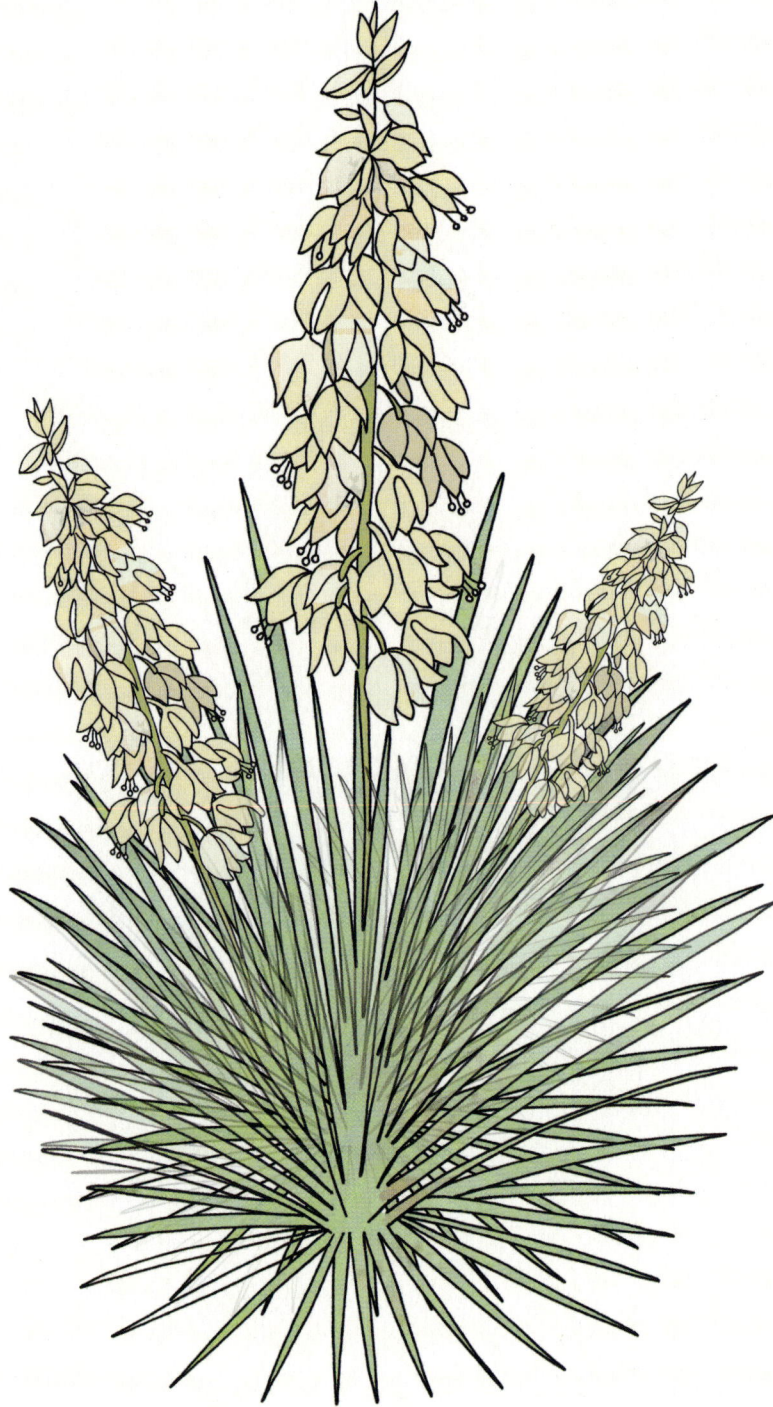

Soaptree Yucca

Yucca elata

Appearance: This tall, spiky, treelike plant is another desert mainstay. Soaptree yuccas can grow up to 20 feet (6 m) tall with fine, pointed, blue-green leaves. They can develop several heads on their trunk-like stem with age. They can sometimes resemble small palm trees. A powerful flowering stem comes out of the top of each head. The flowering stem is covered in creamy-white, succulent-like, bell-shaped flowers. Soaptree yuccas in bloom are truly a sight to see.

Habitat: Sonoran and Mojave Deserts in grasslands and mesas between 1,500 and 6,000 feet (457 and 1,829 m).

Blooming season: April through June.

Lifespan: Can live up to three hundred years.

Environmental roles: Soaptree yuccas provide shelter for small mammals and birds, and host specific yucca moth species that are essential for pollinating the soaptree yucca. This plant is hardy, long-living, and drought tolerant, making it a great option for desert landscaping.

Foraging: The soapy material in the roots and trunks can be used as a soap substitute (thus its name). Its flowers are edible and actually very tasty. The flowers can be eaten raw in salads or they can be fried. They are especially tasty when put in an air fryer. The sooner they are consumed after picking, the better.

Plant friends: Blue yucca and Joshua tree.

Southwestern Prickly Poppy

Argemone pleiacantha

Appearance: This is one of my favorite desert wildflowers because of its soft, fluttery, white petals juxtaposed against its sharp, spiny stems and leaves. It grows erect up to 4 feet (1.2 m) tall and its spiny buds, stems and leaves are a bluish-green color. Its attractive white flowers, 3 inches (7.5 cm) wide, usually have six petals and a dark yellow center. Southwestern prickly poppy is rare and its appearance is unlike any other desert wildflower.

Habitat: Is only found in Arizona, New Mexico, and Northwestern Mexico between 1,500 and 5,000 feet (457 and 1,524 m) elevation in washes, disturbed soils, slopes, and roadsides.

Blooming season: Throughout the whole year but I have found they are happiest in early summer.

Lifespan: Seven to nine years.

Environmental roles: These wildflowers are extremely drought tolerant and can go dormant until conditions are right for them to grow again. They do well in disturbed soils and are often one of the first to grow in a disturbed area. They are great for native pollinators because they produce a lot of pollen and have attractive flowers. They also have deep taproots which help prevent soil erosion. Indigenous peoples have used prickly poppies for a variety of medicinal purposes.

Foraging: This plant has a history of external applications for sores, burns, wounds, etc., but has toxic compounds, so it is not recommended for herbal use.

Plant friends: Sonoran prickly poppy and Mexican prickly poppy.

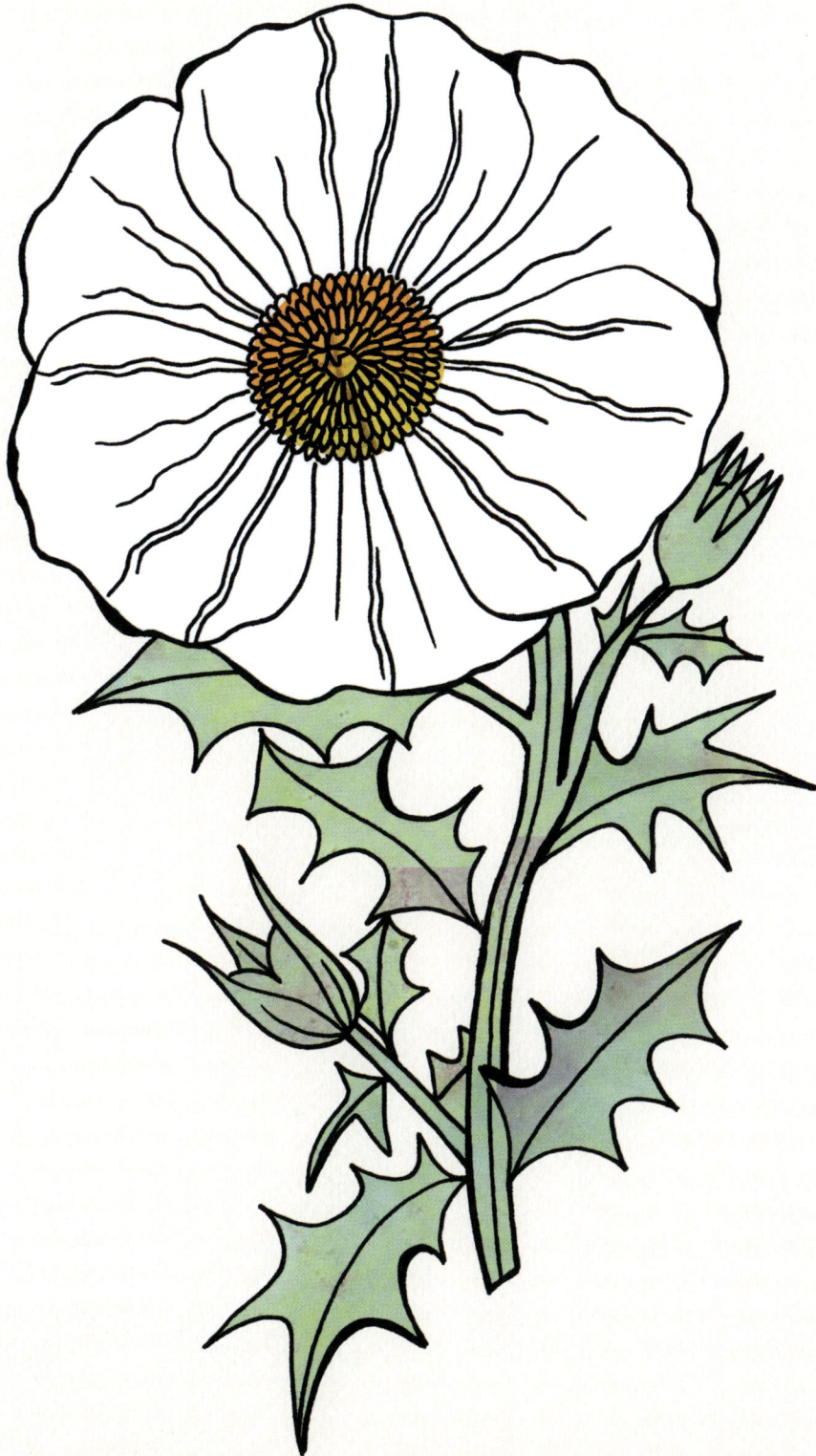

Autumn

The Desert Dries Up

September through November

Fall in the Sonoran Desert always takes us by surprise. After months of oppressive summer heat, we forget what comfort feels like. Then, suddenly, temperatures drop. In the crisp morning air, we remember that everything is cyclical. As the sun's path lowers across the sky, the days get shorter—but the light reaches further, illuminating the landscape in a fresh way, revealing what we could not see before.

Now, many plants go dormant, and the monsoon rains dissipate. Life, so recently replenished, starts to dry out, holding on to the reserves it's built up. Lush green grasses fade to shades of gold while shrubs and trees softly shed their leaves. This transformation is especially stunning in riparian areas where the changing leaves of tall cottonwood and sycamore trees create vibrant ribbons of yellow, copper, and rust across the terrain. This colorful display against the cloudless, azure sky is an exaltation of the shifting seasons, a celebration of change. There is beauty in letting go and surrendering to the softness of autumn. Fall is a season to make space for all that lies ahead.

Autumn always offers me a bit of sorrow. I am always a little sad to see spring and summer go because of the abundance of life they offer, but the cooling temperatures provide a soft respite from the heat. Autumn is a dry season in the Sonoran Desert. The plant life is satiated with plenty of water reserves, and it waits patiently throughout autumn until the winter rain comes. The desert plants are well adapted to this wait and are ready to soak everything up when it finally does rain again. September still feels like summer, with highs around 100°F (38°C), but in mid- to late October, the temperatures start to cool, with chilly mornings and warm afternoons. The leaves start to change color in our sky islands, and a lot of lower desert plants dry up and seed, spreading their essence for the growth of tomorrow. Most desert dwellers who can't handle the heat of other seasons start to spend more time outdoors as the region becomes more temperate. For small business owners in Tucson like myself, autumn marks the busy season when we start to think about the holidays. I love walking along the banks of rivers and finding sunflowers in full bloom during this time. Even as the vitality of the desert dwindles, we're still surrounded by its beauty.

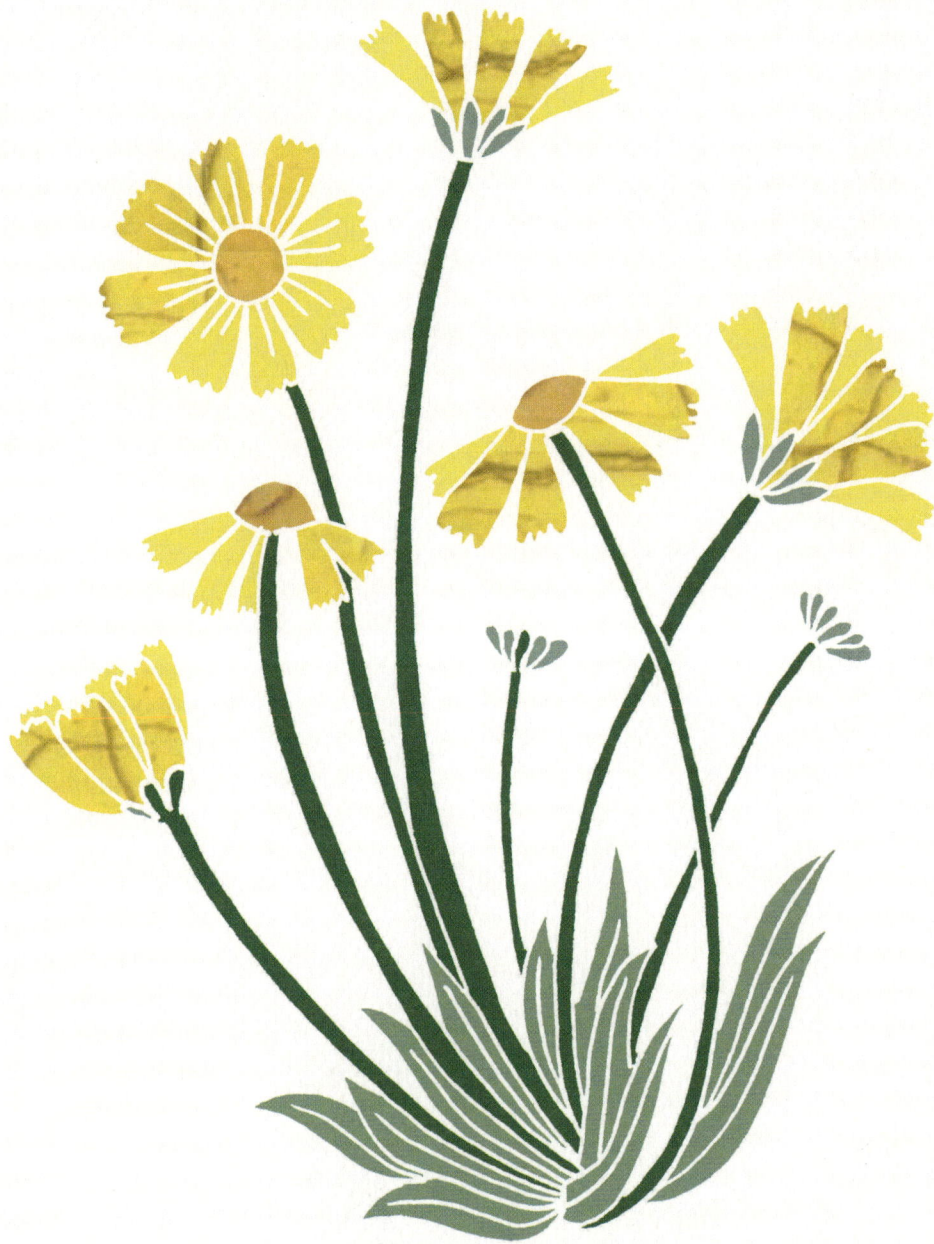

Angelita Daisy

Tetraneuris acaulis

Appearance: This densely tufted, smaller wildflower grows a dark-green bushy base with long flower stems that reach out above it. The whole plant grows no more than 1 foot (30.5 cm) tall and 3 to 5 feet (1 to 1.5 m) wide. It has bright-yellow, daisylike disc-shaped flowers about 2 inches (5 cm) in diameter.

Habitat: Widespread throughout the Western United States. Grows in well-draining, rocky soil. Lower desert to grassland distribution.

Blooming season: This beauty can bloom all year but is most prevalent in the spring and fall here in the desert.

Lifespan: Perennial, three to four years.

Environmental role: This nontoxic, herbaceous wildflower attracts pollinating insects, and is resistant to rabbits and deer. Because it thrives in well-draining, rocky areas, it is great for desert landscaping.

Foraging: I love to use this wildflower in both dried and fresh flower arrangements. It is great for pressing as well. The medicinal properties of this plant are not well known but like many other daisy varieties, it could have some benefits for the skin, inflammatory issues, or stomach ailments. Native Hopi used this wildflower to make a stimulating drink and relieve hip and back pain in pregnant women.

Plant friends: This is another Asteraceae family member, so it has many daisy friends like the blackfoot daisy, desert marigold, and desert aster.

Arizona Fescue Grass

Festuca arizonica

Appearance: This is a tall native grass with rough, blue-green, string-shaped blades which can measure up to 10 inches (25 cm) long. It grows a panicle inflorescence (a group or cluster of flowers arranged on a stem on a main branch). It produces seeds at the end of the inflorescence stems.

Habitat: Grows in the lower Southwestern United States and is usually found in larger stands in higher elevations of 6,000 to 10,000 feet (1,829 to 3,048 m) above sea level. Found in dry, shallow clay soils and sandy to gravelly soils.

Blooming season: Remains green from summer to autumn.

Lifespan: Perennial and can lie dormant through drought periods.

Environmental role: Arizona fescue grass has a fibrous root system that is great for erosion control. It flourishes on roadsides and in yards. The seeds it produces are a wonderful food source for local birds. The grass itself is grazed on by deer, elk, antelope, and bighorn sheep. It enjoys full sun and is drought tolerant, making it a perfect fit for Arizona. It also provides great ground coverage for smaller wildlife.

Foraging: No medicinal properties known but it looks nice in dried autumn arrangements.

Plant friends: Other types of grass like mountain muhly and blue grama often grow next to Arizona fescue.

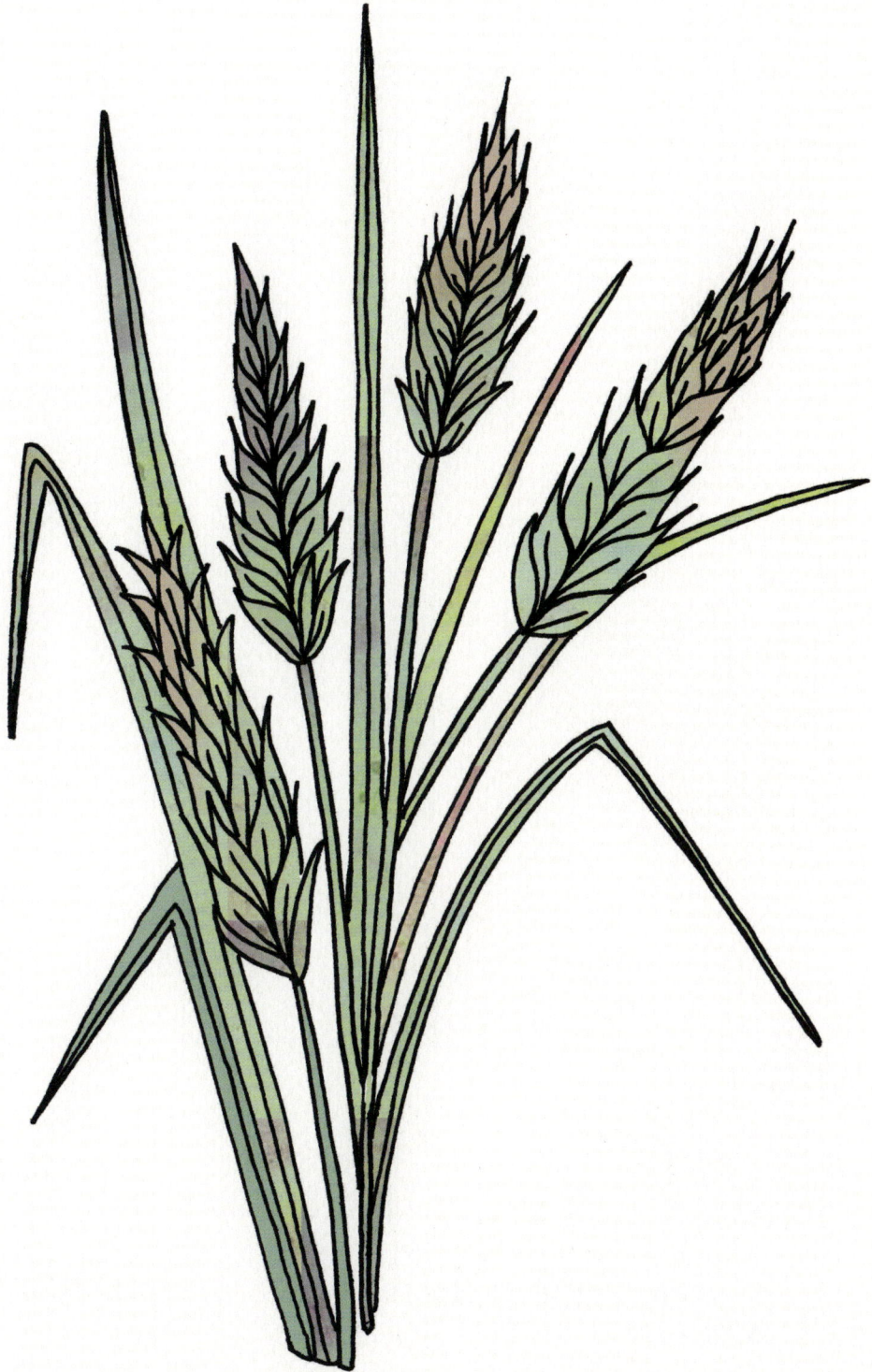

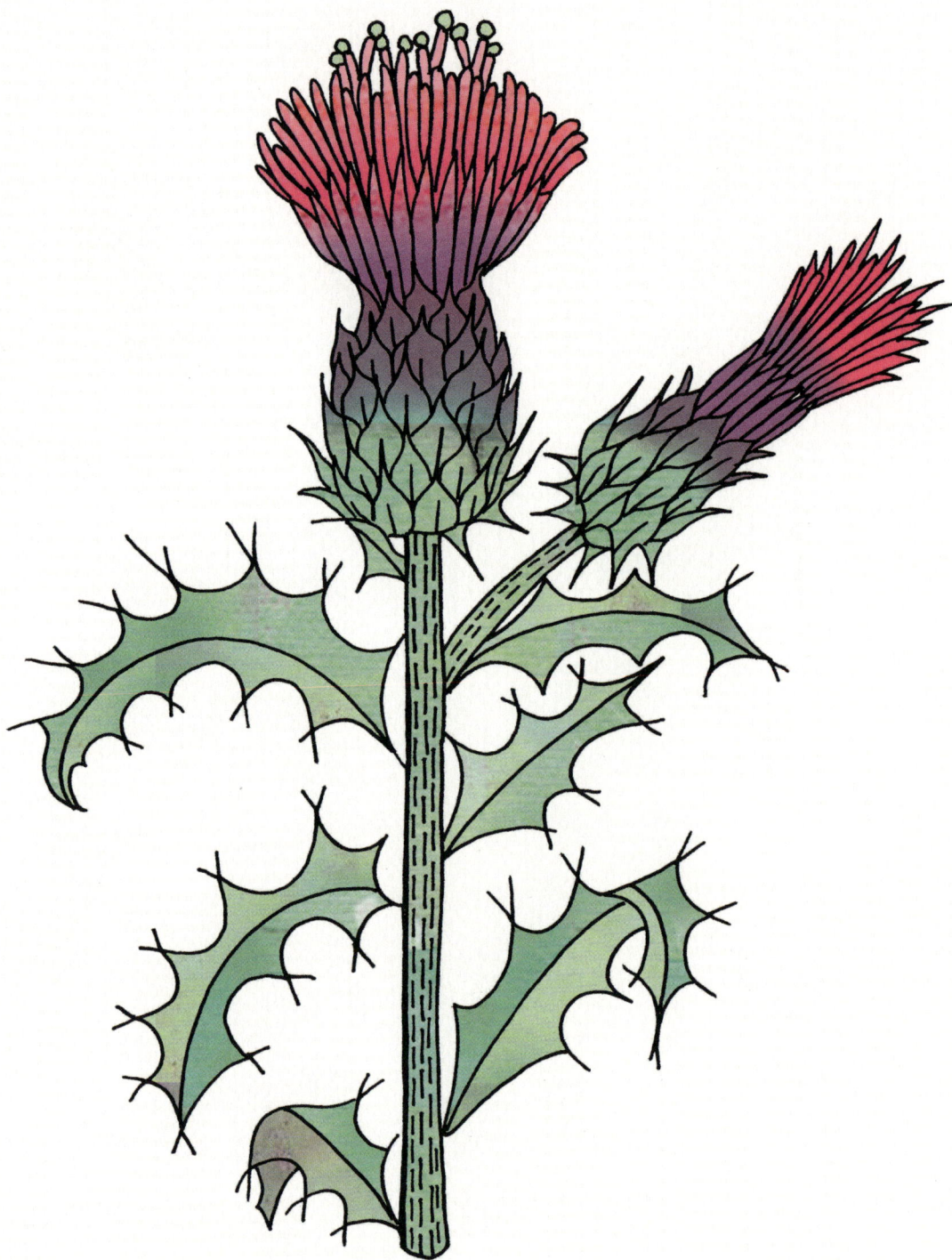

Arizona Thistle

Cirsium arizonicum

Appearance: These spiny wildflowers are a true desert being. They have grayish, hairy, erect stems and long grayish-green, triangular, pointed leaves covered in sharp spines. These plants can grow up to 5 feet (1.5 m) tall. They have multiple bright-red flower heads at the end of one stem, each growing up to 2 inches (5 cm) long. Each flower head has small, straight, clustered petals with many spines surrounding the base. The flower heads never look fully open, unlike other rounded thistle heads. These spiky fellas are both beautiful and defensive, like many desert plants.

Habitat: Southwestern United States and Northwestern Mexico in mountain ranges, grasslands, and woodlands between 3,000 and 9,500 feet (914 and 2,896 m) elevation.

Blooming season: May through October.

Lifespan: Depending on the weather and where it is growing, Arizona thistle can be either a biennial plant (living up to two years to complete its full life cycle) or perennial (living longer than two years).

Environmental role: Arizona thistles play an important role in the high desert because their blooming season is a little longer than other wildflowers'. They provide nectar and pollen for insects, and their leaves, seeds, and pollen are food sources for moth and butterfly larvae (important pollinators). The seeds are rich in nutrients and are an important dietary staple for wild birds.

Foraging: No known uses for foraging.

Plant friends: New Mexico thistle and bull thistle.

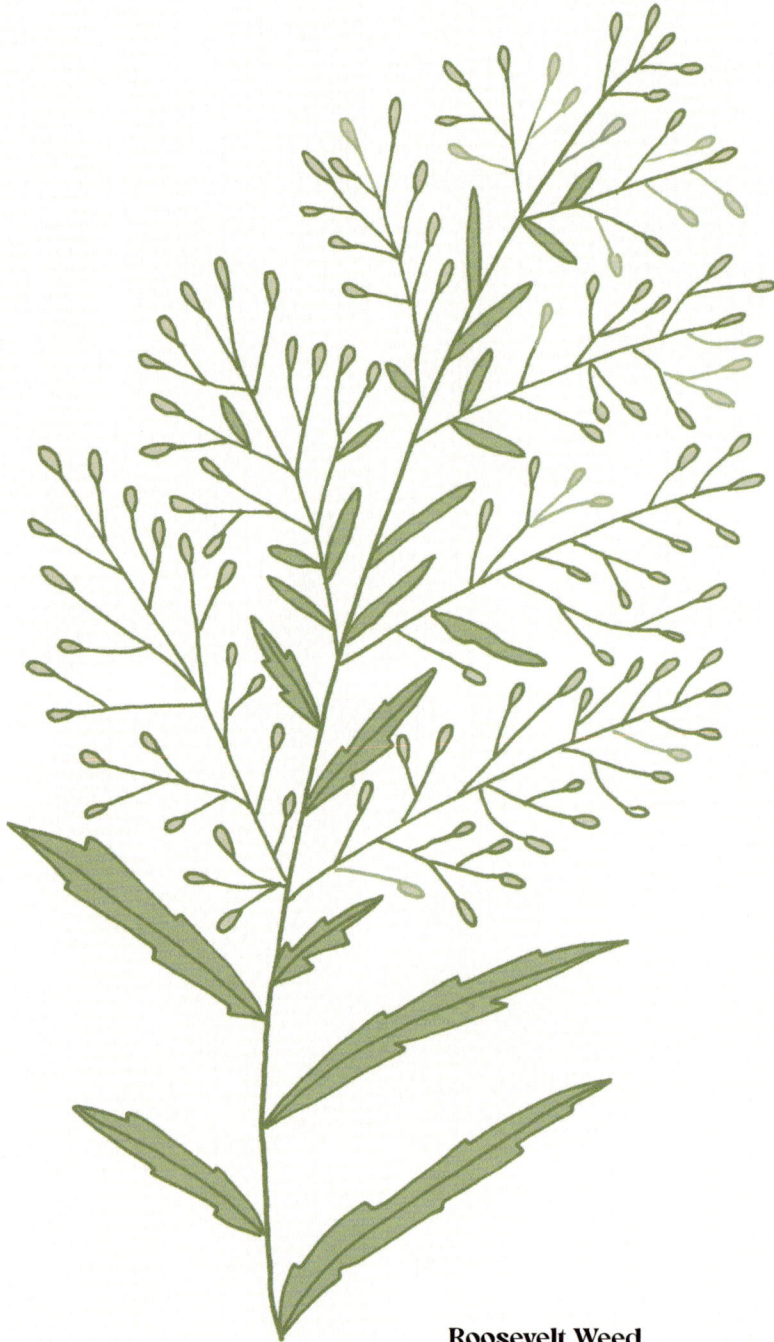

Roosevelt Weed

Baccharis: Desert Broom and Roosevelt Weed

Baccharis sarothroides / Baccharis neglecta

I will be talking about these two native plants together as they are very similar to each other and are found growing in the same habitats.

Appearance: Both are hardy shrubs. Desert broom can grow as tall as 10 feet (3 m) whereas Roosevelt weed can grow up to 14 feet (4 m). Both male and female flowers grow on separate plants, which makes the flowers appear different from plant to plant. The flower plumes are distinctive with soft, small, greenish-white heads. They both have small, thin, bright-green leaves. They both produce fluffy fruits (which contain the seed) but desert broom is known for the way its fruit becomes airborne and covers the surrounding area with a beautiful, white, snow-like blanket.

Habitat: Desert and grassland biomes as well as riparian communities between 1,000 and 5,500 feet (305 and 1,676 m), but mostly lower deserts with gravel or sandy washes. They are tenacious and can easily grow in disturbed areas like saline soil, roadsides, and flood plains. While desert broom and Roosevelt weed are both found in the Southwest, the latter can also be found as far east as North Carolina.

Blooming season: August through November (sometimes through February).

Lifespan: Perennial, ten to twenty years.

Environmental role: Both of these plants have thick fibrous roots that can help prevent erosion in riparian areas. Because they can grow well in neglected places, they are great for native landscaping in parking lots or roadsides. They both spread their seed far and wide, easily taking over patches of land.

Foraging: Roosevelt weed is said to be toxic, but desert broom has many medicinal uses. The leaves and stems can be used to make tea to treat colds and sinus issues. Topically it can be used to relieve sore muscles. See the following page for a tincture recipe.

Plant friends: Roosevelt weed and desert broom are definitely besties. Seepwillow (also called mule fat) often grows near these two and is also a Baccharis.

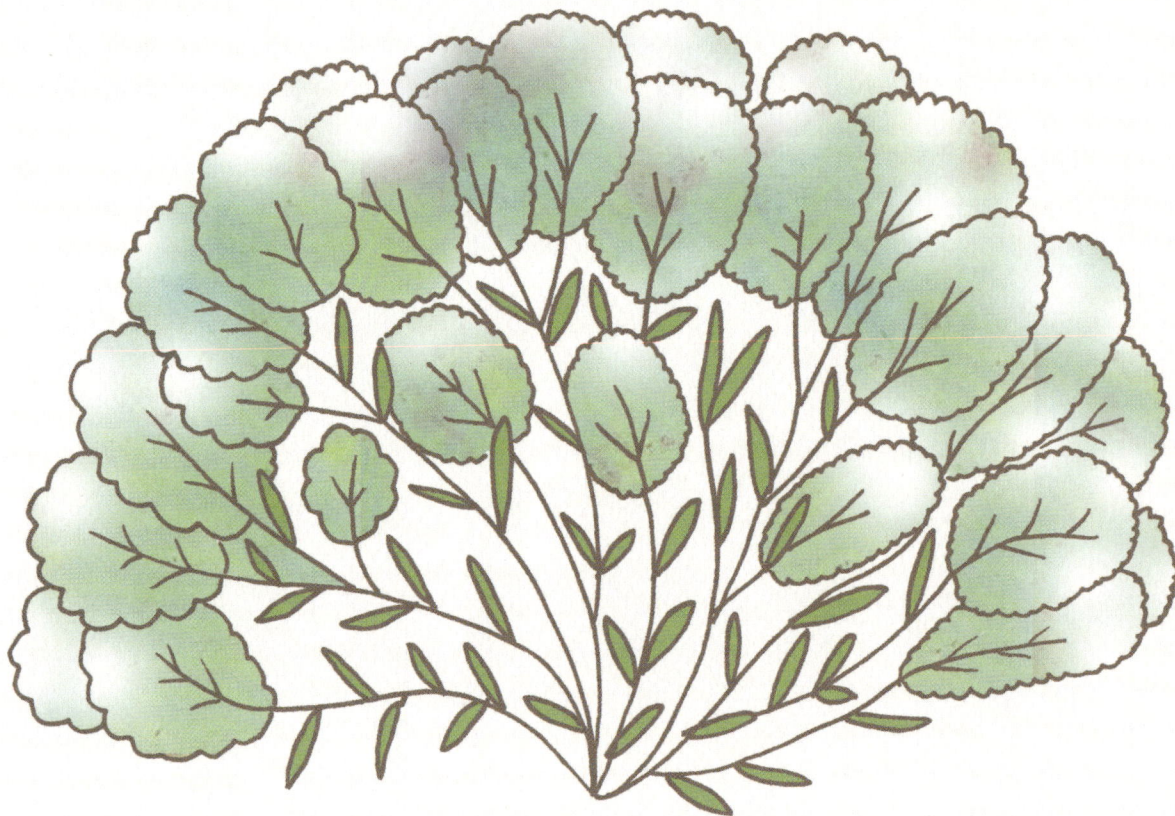

Desert Broom

Desert Broom Tincture

This tincture is great to make now as cooler weather can bring on more colds and sinus congestion. It will help soothe colds and other aching ailments. Desert broom has anti-inflammatory and cholesterol-lowering capabilities as well as antioxidants.

MATERIALS

- A few foraged desert broom branches with plenty of green leaves on them (make sure to take them from a safe space, away from roadsides or street water runoff)

- Paper bag (optional)

- Scissors

- 16-ounce (0.5 L) sterilized glass jar with lid

- 1 quart (1 L) Everclear (grain alcohol) or vodka

- Strainer

- Dropper bottle

INSTRUCTIONS

1. Let the branches dry out in the open (they can be placed in a paper, but not plastic, bag if desired). Drying can take anywhere between 1 and 3 weeks depending on the moisture in the environment.

2. Remove all the green leaves from the main stems.

3. Using scissors, cut leaves into smaller ½- to 1-inch (1 to 2.5 cm) pieces.

4. Fill the jar almost to the top with the chopped leaves.

5. Pour the Everclear or vodka over the leaves, until the tops of the leaves are just covered.

6. Place the jar in a dark place, such as a cupboard, and let sit for 1 month.

7. After 1 month has passed, strain the liquid and pour it into a dropper bottle.

8. Take 1 or 2 drops orally when you feel a cold coming on or if you already have symptoms. You can also rub this tincture into sore muscles for relief.

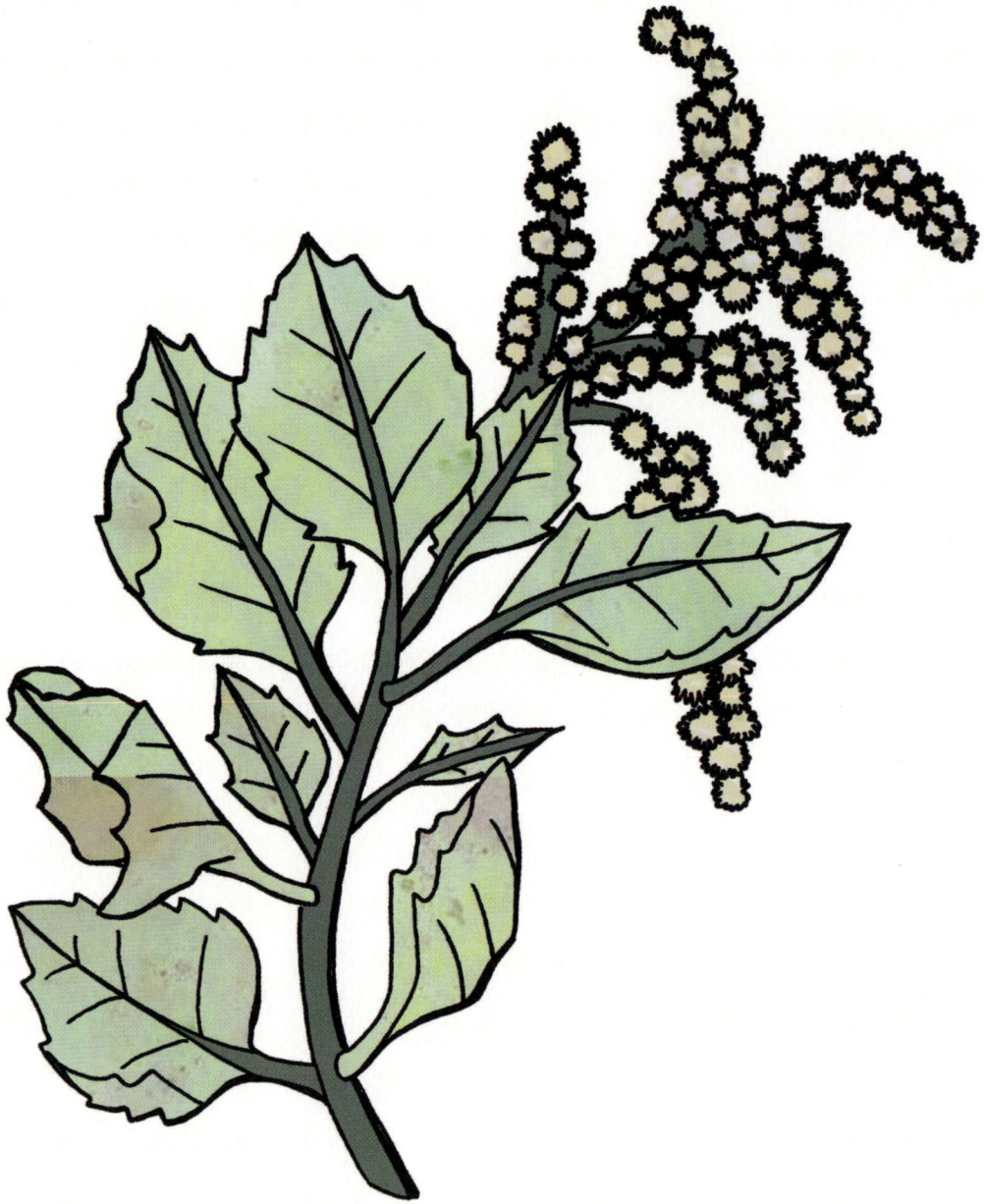

Big Saltbush

Atriplex lentiformis

Appearance: This large, multibranched shrub can reach up to 12 feet (4 m) tall and forms a dense bush with scaly, grayish-green leaves covering its branches. The leaves and stems are covered in dense bladder hairs that excrete salt and give the leaf a silvery sheen. In summer or autumn, it produces cream-colored flowers in tassel-like clusters. This bush is big, unique, and beautiful in autumn.

Habitat: Southwestern United States and Northern Mexico in low-alkaline soils, grasslands, riparian wetlands, marshes, and dry lakes from sea level up to 4,900 feet (1,494 m) elevation.

Blooming season: March through October.

Lifespan: Can live more than one hundred years!

Environmental role: Big saltbush pulls salts from water into its roots and into the tiny hairs on its leaves, meaning it can withstand difficult environments where other desert plants cannot, and providing important cover for desert wildlife to approach water sources. It also continuously provides food for desert wildlife and Indigenous peoples, who have consumed its tiny seeds for thousands of years.

Foraging: The leaves, flowers, and stems can be crushed, steamed, and inhaled to relieve nasal congestion or used as a poultice to treat bug bites. Chewing the fresh leaves can help with head colds. This plant is edible and has a salty taste but is rich in niacin and is best used as a seasoning.

Plant friends: Four-wing saltbush.

California Buckwheat

Eriogonum fasciculatum

Appearance: California buckwheat is a spreading shrub that can bush out up to 6 feet (1.8 m) wide and 3 feet (91 cm) tall. It has small leathery leaves with curled edges. It produces beautiful clusters of cotton-like flowers that range from white to pink and turn a rust color when dried—truly unique beauties. It frequently flowers even through the heat of the summer.

Habitat: Mojave and Sonoran Deserts on dry, rocky slopes and canyons from sea level up to 7,500 feet (2,286 m) elevation.

Blooming season: January through December.

Lifespan: Can live up to fifty years.

Environmental role: These hardy bushes play a pivotal role for native pollinators because of their long blooming season. California buckwheat is great for landscaping because it does not require much water and survives through the extreme heat and extreme cold of the desert. It makes great ground cover which can help moisture retention in the soil and gives shelter to smaller wildlife. It produces tiny seeds which feed wildlife and can be ground into a flour and eaten. The Cahuilla people use this plant as a remedy for headaches, stomachaches, and bladder infections.

Foraging: The leaves and flowers of this plant can be used medicinally but I personally love to collect them to add to dried floral arrangements because they retain their structure when dried and have a unique shape.

Plant friends: St. Catherine's lace and Conejo buckwheat.

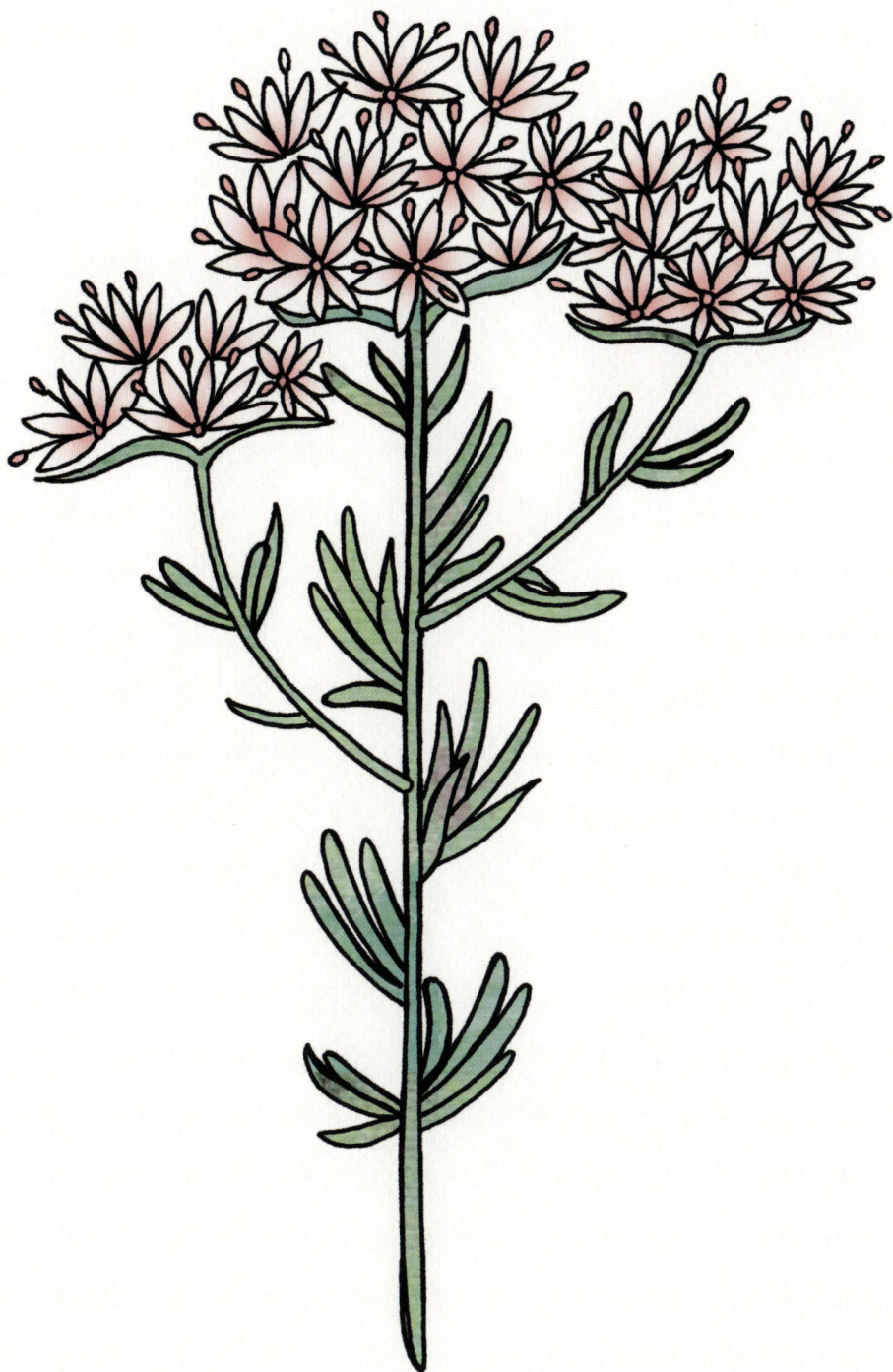

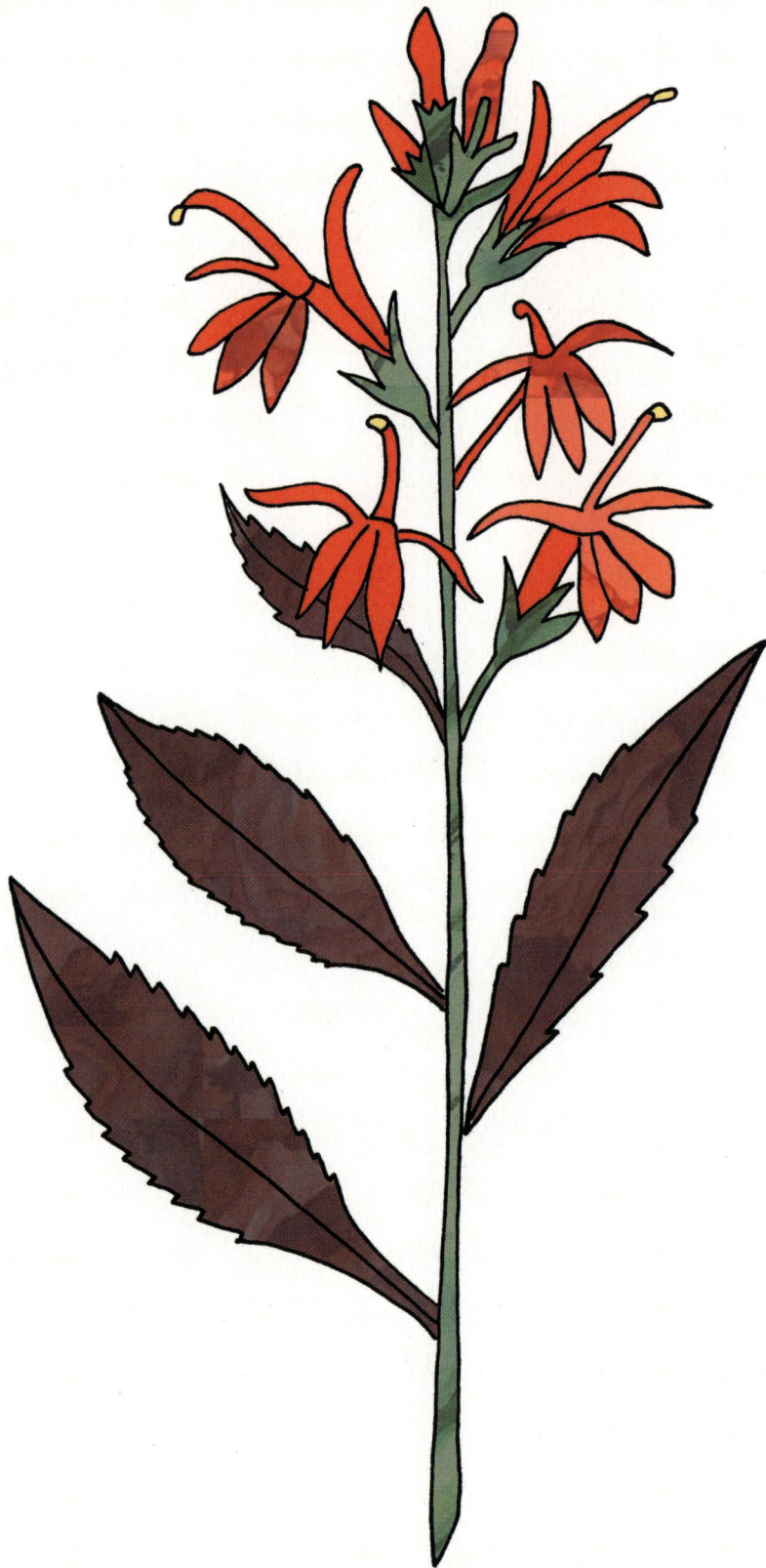

Cardinal Flower

Lobelia cardinalis

Appearance: Cardinal flowers can grow up to 6 feet (1.8 m) tall with long individual spikes that have clusters of bright-red flowers with three spreading lower petals and two upper petals. The stem is lined with thin, dark-green, lance-shaped leaves. These flowers contrast against their green environment and remind me of little decorated flag poles.

Habitat: Found almost all over the United States on wet slopes and stream sides in rich soil. However, it is rare in Arizona, found mostly in the sky island regions.

Blooming season: July through September.

Lifespan: Short-lived, up to two years.

Environmental role: The cardinal flower's bright-red, slightly tubular flowers produce nectar that hummingbirds are very attracted to. It is self-sowing, so it can replenish its population.

Foraging: The Iroquois have used its leaves and roots to help with fevers, colds, and stomachaches but this plant, like many medicines, can be toxic if eaten in large quantities. This plant isn't very common in Arizona, so I suggest letting it be.

Plant friends: Sierra Madre lobelia.

Catclaw Acacia

Senegalia greggii

Appearance: Catclaw acacia is sometimes treelike, growing up to 20 feet (6 m) tall, but it is actually a rounded shrub that averages 5 feet (1.5 m) tall. It has many branches that are covered with catclaw–shaped thorns and tiny, rounded, gray-green leaves. The fragrant flowers are fluffy and bushy and form 2-inch (5 cm) spikes. I love the way acacia flowers smell: slightly sweet with a soapy tinge. These plants also produce slightly twisted pealike pods that are seen hanging from their branches in autumn.

Habitat: Mojave, Sonoran, and Chihuahuan Deserts in chaparral and brushlands or along washes and banks in caliche (clay), sandy, or rocky soils between 360 feet and 4,600 feet (110 m and 1,402 m) elevation.

Blooming season: April through October.

Lifespan: Can live up to 120 years old.

Environmental role: Catclaw acacia is very common throughout the Sonoran Desert and makes terrain difficult to traverse because of its sharp thorns and wiry branches. It plays a crucial role in preventing soil erosion and protecting small wildlife from larger predators, and its hardwood can create long-lasting tools and firewood. It is of special importance to honeybees and native bees because the flowers produce sugar-rich nectar (I have tasted catclaw honey and it is delicious). Ants also use this nectar as a food source.

Foraging: This shrub has many uses! The pods of catclaw acacia can be eaten fresh or dried and ground into flour for baking. The pods can also be used to make an eyewash to treat conjunctivitis. The leaves are good for making a tea that soothes sore throats. Native Southwestern peoples use the wood to create fibers, firewood, and building material. It has many more uses and is prevalent in the Southwest so can be foraged easily.

Plant friends: Sweet acacia, palo verde trees.

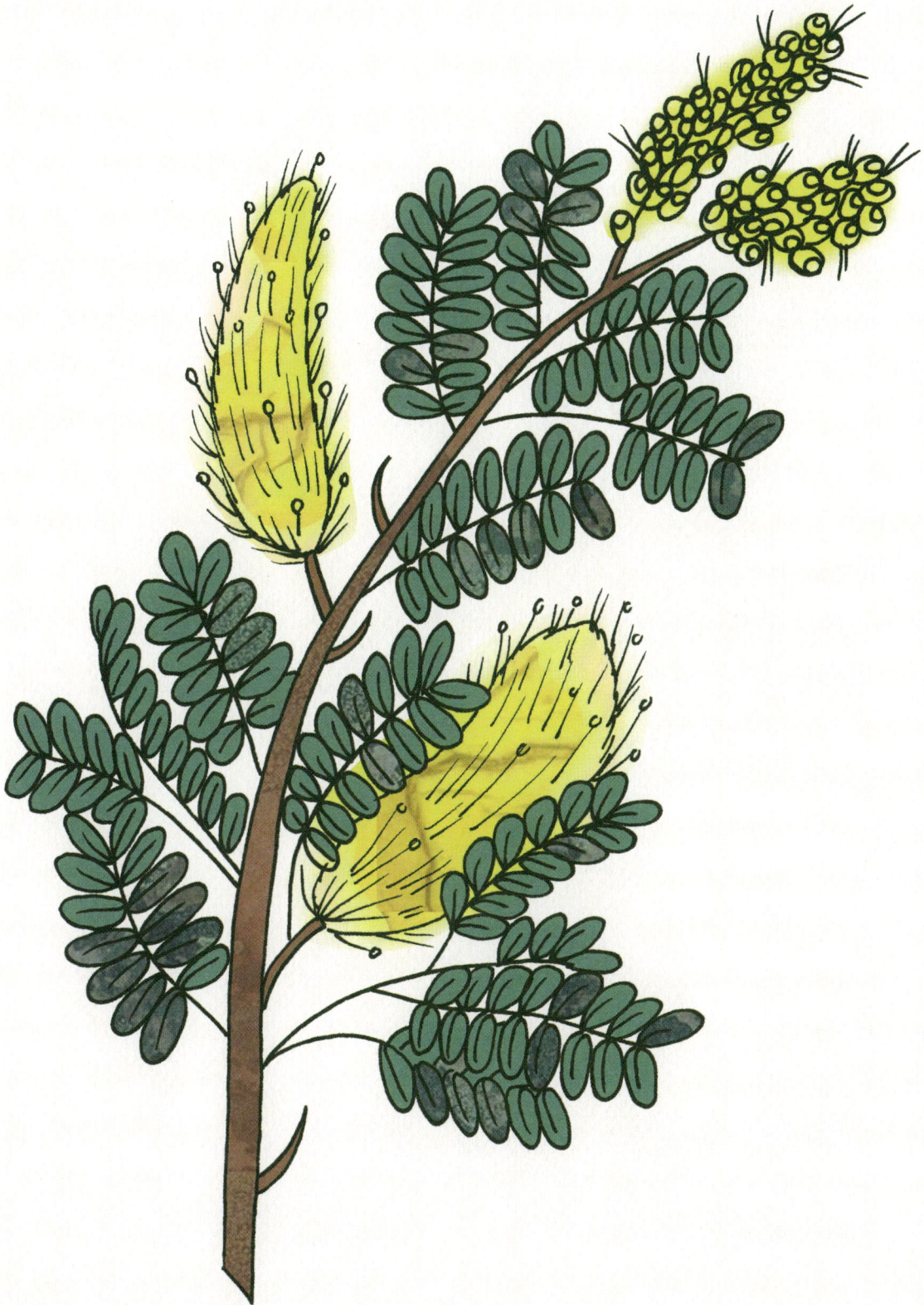

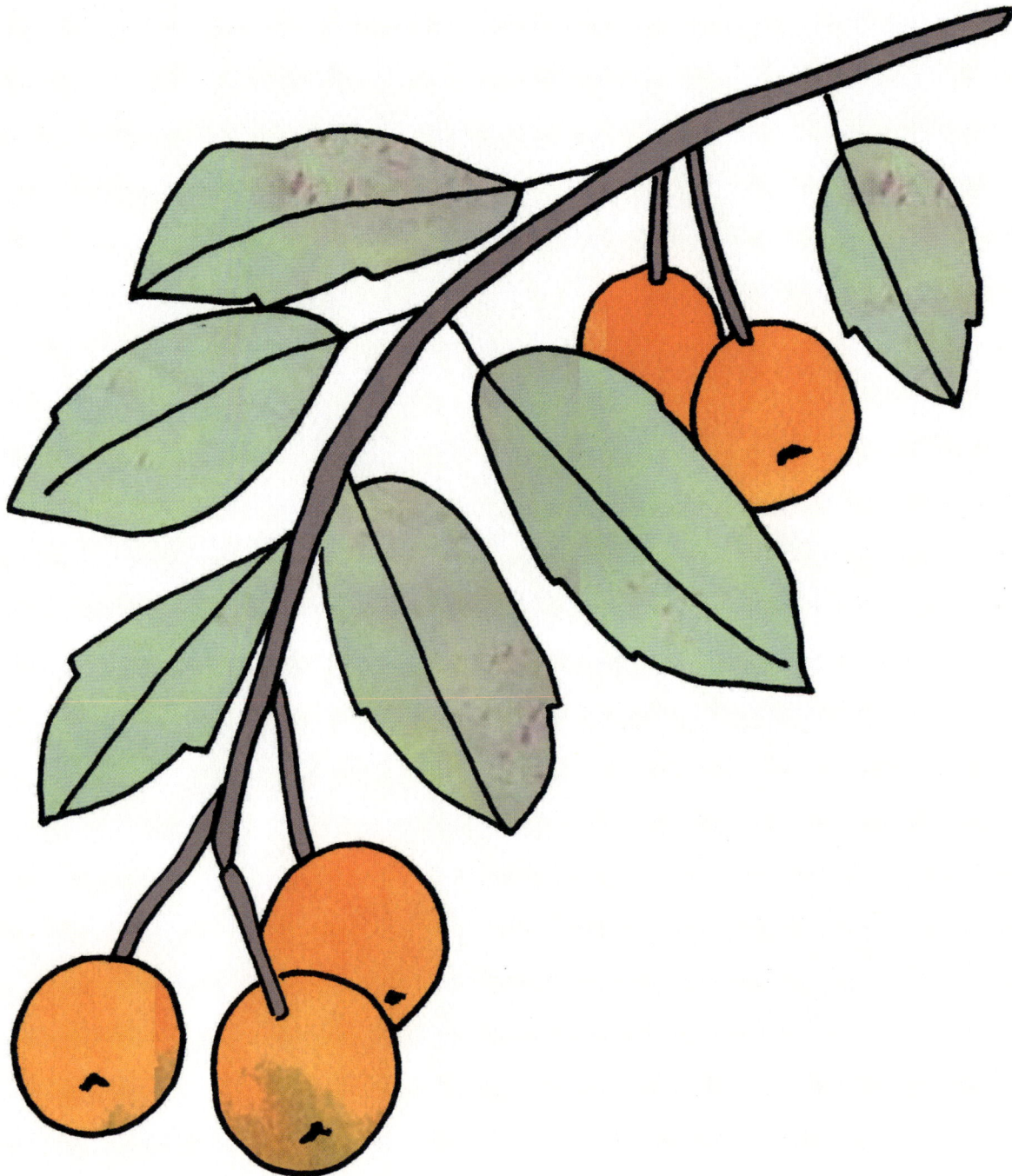

Desert Hackberry

Celtis ehrenbergiana

Appearance: Desert hackberry is a favorite of mine as it is pretty common in southern Arizona. It is a thorny, scraggly shrub (like many Sonoran Desert plants) with zigzagging branches that have a grayish bark. It can grow as tall as 15 feet (5 m) and has small, oval, bright-green (sometimes toothed) leaves. It blooms clusters of small white flowers in late spring and early summer which then fruit into bright yellowish-orange edible berries that will cover the bush in autumn.

Habitat: Southern Arizona and southern Texas between elevations of 1,000 and 4,000 feet (305 and 1,219 m). Most commonly found in and around washes or in mesquite bosques (groves of close growing mesquite trees).

Blooming season: February through May.

Fruiting season: September through October (in southern Arizona).

Lifespan: Can live up to one thousand years old! (Now this is unbelievable!)

Environmental role: Desert hackberry berries are a pivotal food source for so many desert animals, including humans, because they are so rich in nutrients. Its flowers are important for native pollinators and its root systems prevent soil erosion. Its dense, thorny branches provide shelter and shade for small animals as well.

Foraging: Desert hackberry berries are one of my favorite desert foods to forage. They are distinct, easy to spot, tasty, and provide crude protein, natural sugars, and fiber. I like to eat them raw as is, on top of salads and desserts, or incorporated in baked goods. Each plant offers a slightly different-tasting berry, so tasting while foraging is a must. Be sure to leave plenty behind for wildlife.

Plant friends: Netleaf hackberry, common hackberry.

Desert Milkweed

Asclepias subulata

Appearance: These succulent-like plants are very striking. They have tall, often leafless, greenish-white stems that can grow up to 9 feet (2.7 m) tall with unique, light yellowish-green umbel (umbrella-shaped) flowers at the tips of the stems. They can grow small linear leaves after adequate rainfall and the flowers fruit to narrow, smooth pods 2 to 4 inches (5 to 10 cm) long.

Habitat: The Sonoran Desert on dry slopes, mesas, and washes up to 3,000 feet (914 m) elevation.

Blooming season: April through December.

Lifespan: Can live up to ten years.

Environmental role: This plant is well adapted to the harsh desert environment and is of special value to pollinators like the monarch butterfly and queen butterfly as well as honeybees. Desert milkweed has been an important medicinal plant to Indigenous peoples over time.

Foraging: The sap from the desert milkweed can be toxic to humans and animals. However, the Seri people have used the roots for headaches, toothaches, and heart problems. Proceed with caution and research if you use this plant medicinally. This plant is beneficial to pollinators, so it is probably best left alone.

Plant friends: Pineneedle milkweed and Arizona milkweed.

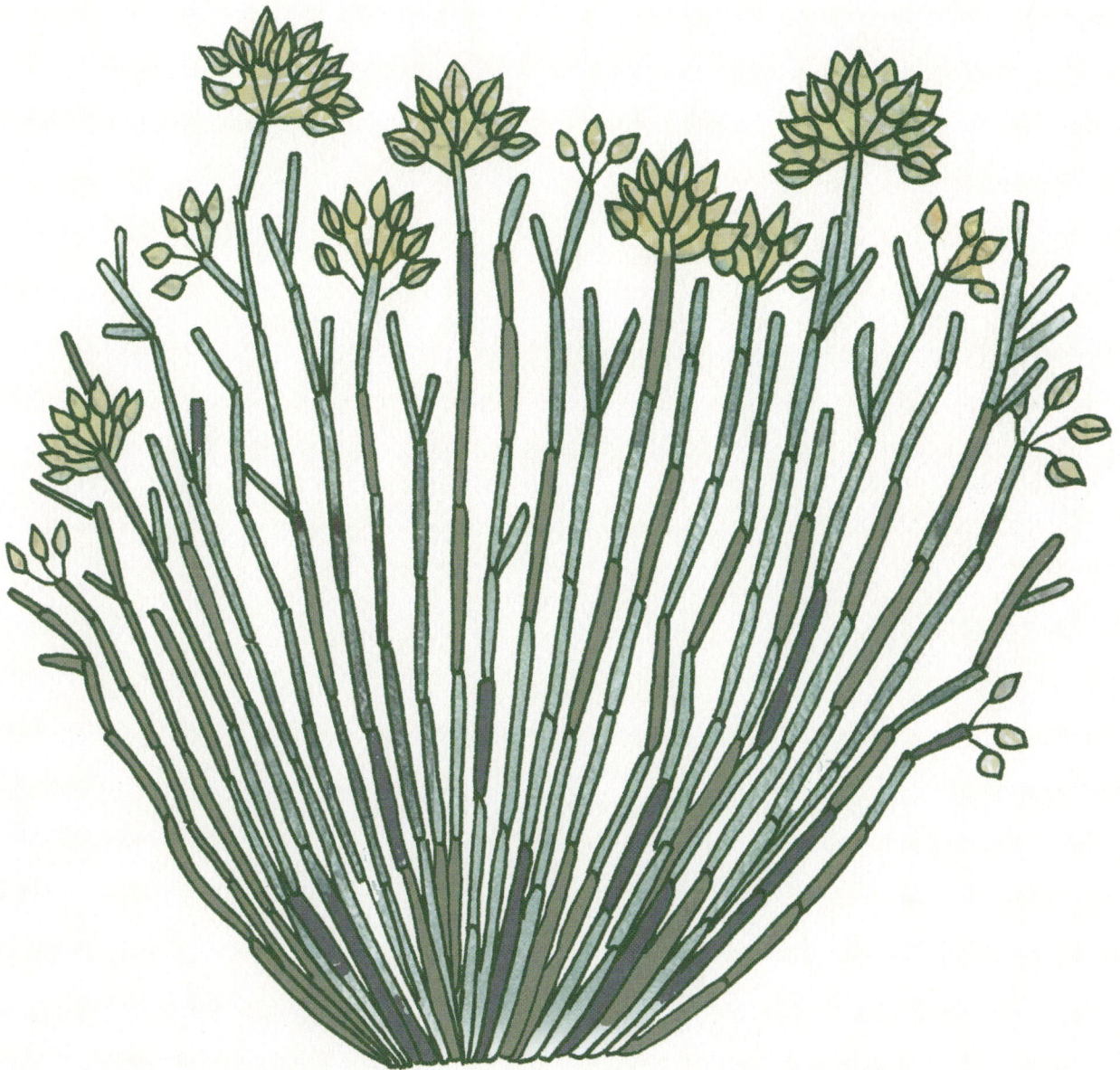

Fishhook Barrel Cactus

Ferocactus wislizeni

Appearance: These iconic thick, barrel-shaped cacti are covered in long, hooked spines and are usually about 5 feet (1.5 m) tall, but can be bigger. Gorgeous, bright yellow to red flowers bloom at the circular top of the cactus; they're 3 inches (7.5 cm) across and have a waxy look and feel to them. In autumn the flowers dry and are replaced with yellow, spineless, barrel-shaped edible fruit that is filled with electrolytes and poppy-like seeds.

Habitat: The Sonoran and Chihuahuan Deserts in desert grassland and rocky areas between 1,000 and 5,300 feet (305 and 1,615 m) elevation.

Blooming season: June through November (in southern Arizona the blooms are most prominent July through September).

Lifespan: Can live up to 130 years.

Environmental role: The fishhook barrel cactus is essential to the ecosystem of the Sonoran Desert. Its fruit provides food to many desert animals and its stored water can be a source of hydration in times of drought. Native peoples of the Sonoran Desert also use its fruit to make candy and jelly. The flowers produce pollen, an important food source for bees.

Foraging: The fishhook barrel cactus fruit is high in vitamins A and C. It has a slightly sour taste but can be eaten raw, used fresh in salsa, cooked into jams, chutney, or jelly, or incorporated in baked goods. The seeds can be dried and ground into flour or added whole into breads, cereals, soups, and more. The fruit is best used when ripe: it will be all yellow with no green left. Only forage a couple of fruits from each barrel, and leave the majority for wildlife. A few fruits go a long way. The spines can also be heated and bent to use as fishhooks (thus its name).

Plant friends: Golden barrel cactus.

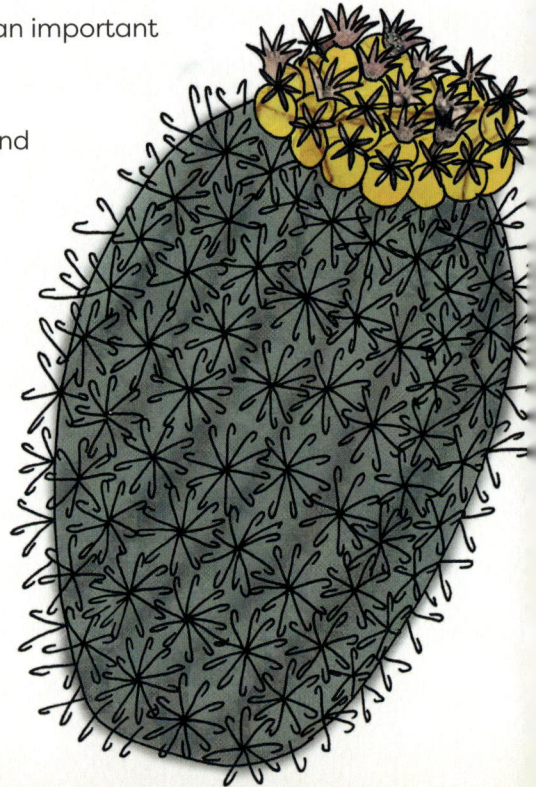

Barrel Cactus Fruit Avocado Pico

INGREDIENTS

- 4 ripe barrel cactus fruits
- 2 plum tomatoes, diced
- 2 avocados (not overly ripe), diced
- ¼ white onion, diced
- 1 serrano chile (optional)
- 6 sprigs cilantro, finely chopped
- 1 teaspoon sea salt
- Juice of 1 lime

INSTRUCTIONS

1. Remove and discard the very top of the barrel cactus fruit, including the dried flowers, then rinse the fruit.

2. Dice the fruit into small ¼-inch (6 mm) pieces (keep the seeds with the diced fruit; they will be included).

3. Remove the stem, seeds, and veins of the chile, then finely chop.

4. Place all ingredients into a medium bowl and mix well.

5. Cover and refrigerate for 30 minutes to let the flavors blend.

6. Serve with chips as a dip or as topping for tacos or other meals.

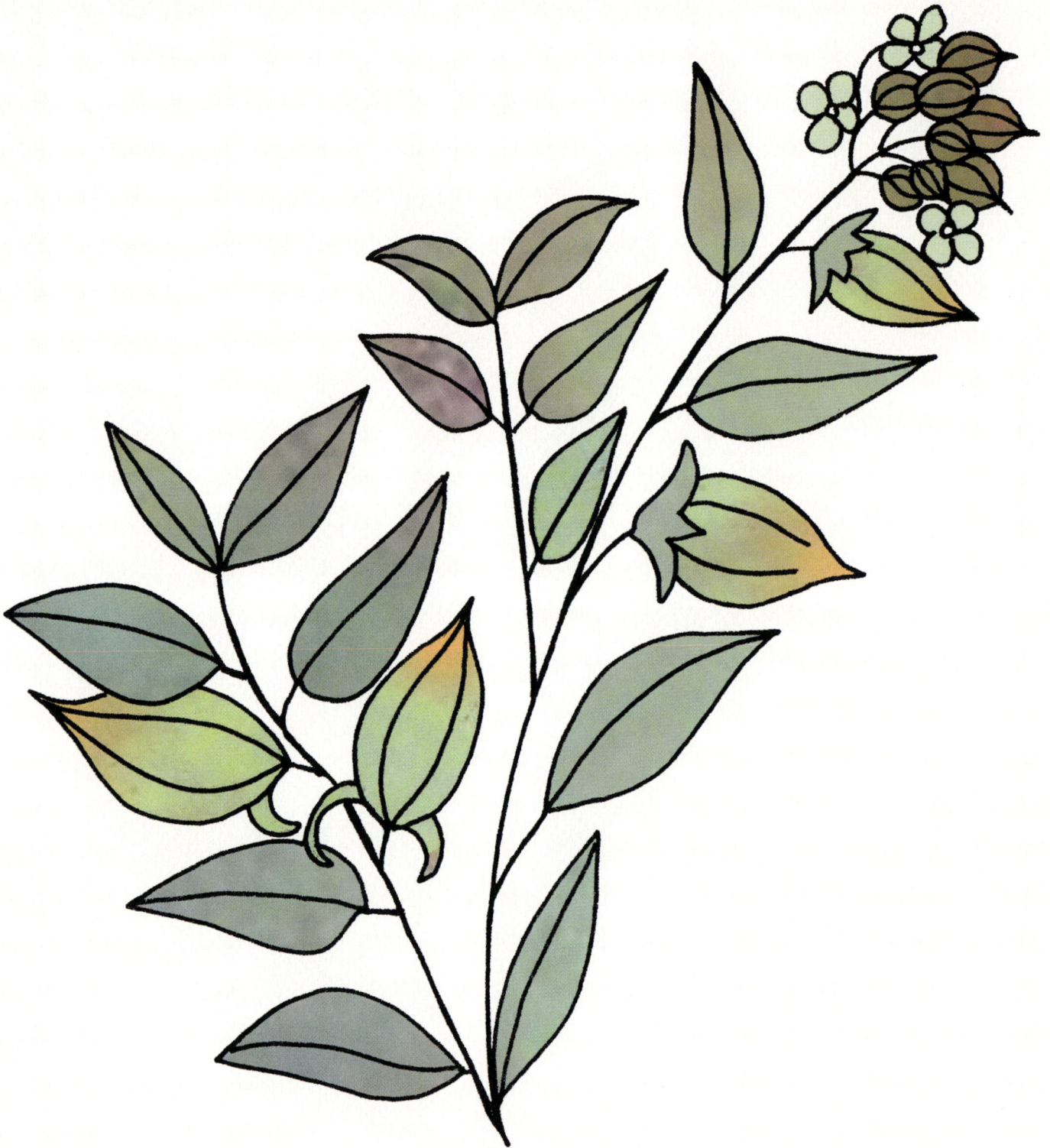

Jojoba

Simmondsia chinensis

Appearance: This evergreen, desert shrub is vital to the Sonoran Desert and is a personal favorite of mine because of the importance of jojoba seed oil in the desert skincare creations I make. This handsome plant, often mistaken for a tree, can grow up to 6 feet (1.8 m) tall with multiple branches that are covered in oval-shaped, bluish-green leaves. The flowers are yellow and grow in small clusters that hang off the stem of the branches. Each flower then fruits into an oval-shaped, acorn-like seed. The seed pods can be up to 1½ inches (4 cm) long. Originally green, once dried they have a light brown shell that contains an edible dark-brown nut.

Habitat: The Sonoran and Mojave Deserts along dry slopes and washes between 1,000 and 5,000 feet (305 and 1,524 m) elevation.

Blooming season: December through March with the seeds ripening in the summer.

Lifespan: Can live up to two hundred years.

Environmental role: The jojoba's long lifespan creates an important, continuous food source for desert wildlife and humans, offering its nuts in the summer every year. It offers shelter to many small desert animals. Jojoba is drought resistant and helps prevent land degradation in dry areas, making it a great plant for xeriscaping (desert landscaping). Jojoba plants are often grown for their seeds, which produce oil that is high in vitamin E, antioxidants, and anti-aging properties—making it a great natural ingredient in skincare and hair care products. Jojoba oil actually mimics our skin's natural oils.

Foraging: Indigenous peoples and desert wildlife have been consuming jojoba seeds for thousands of years. The jojoba nuts can be eaten raw in small amounts, roasted and ground into a paste to spread (like other nut butters), or made into a coffee-like beverage. The oil can be pressed from the seeds and used in a multitude of beneficial ways. I personally purchase jojoba oil from a local farm instead of foraging to create the oil; to make it at home would take so much foraging that it would not be sustainable for the desert or myself. I do like to munch on the seeds as I hike in the summer and early autumn—they taste like almonds.

Plant friends: Jojoba is the only plant in the Simmondsiaceae family—completely unique!

Mexican Manzanita

Arctostaphylos pungens

Appearance: This fiery shrub stands out against the high-desert landscape with its twisting, thick, reddish-brown stems that look like small tree trunks. Manzanita doesn't look like any other desert shrub and is easily recognizable. It can grow up to 7 feet (2.1 m) tall and has thick, dark-green, oval-shaped leaves. It grows light-pink flower clusters in the spring and fruits a small, reddish, edible berry in late summer through autumn. Manzanita means "little apple" in Spanish—the name refers to its small berries, which taste like and resemble apples.

Habitat: Much of the Southwestern United States on rocky slopes and desert ridges in sandy or gravelly soil between 3,500 and 6,500 feet (1,067 and 1,981 m) elevation (found in the sky islands of the Sonoran Desert).

Blooming season: February through May with berries ripe from July through October.

Lifespan: Can live up to fifty years.

Environmental role: Manzanita are early colonizers after fires because their seeds germinate only after they have been scarified by fire. This is interesting to me as their trunk-like stems resemble the shape of fire, too. They are very drought tolerant and grow in areas that many other plants will not. Their berries provide an important food source for birds and mammals of the high desert, and are full of vitamin C and rich in antioxidants. Their flowers are a nectar source for bees and hummingbirds.

Foraging: Manzanita leaves can be chewed into a poultice that can treat open sores, headaches, and ease stomach cramping. Their berries are tasty, slightly sweet, and a little grainy, almost like a tiny apple. Their seeds are very hard so it's probably best not to eat those. I like the berries as a tasty trail snack but I am sure they could be incorporated into all kinds of meals.

Plant friends: Pringle manzanita and greenleaf manzanita.

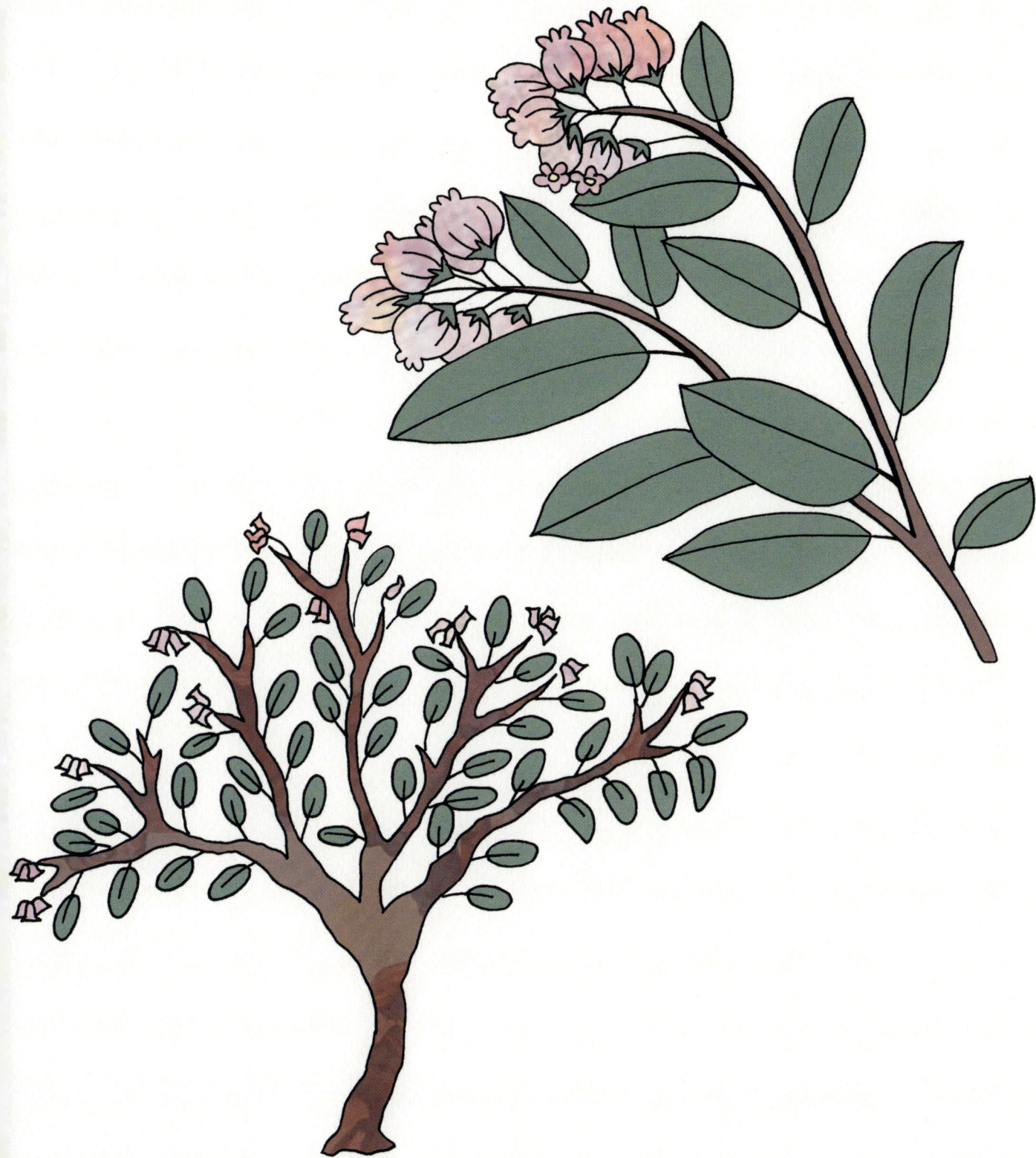

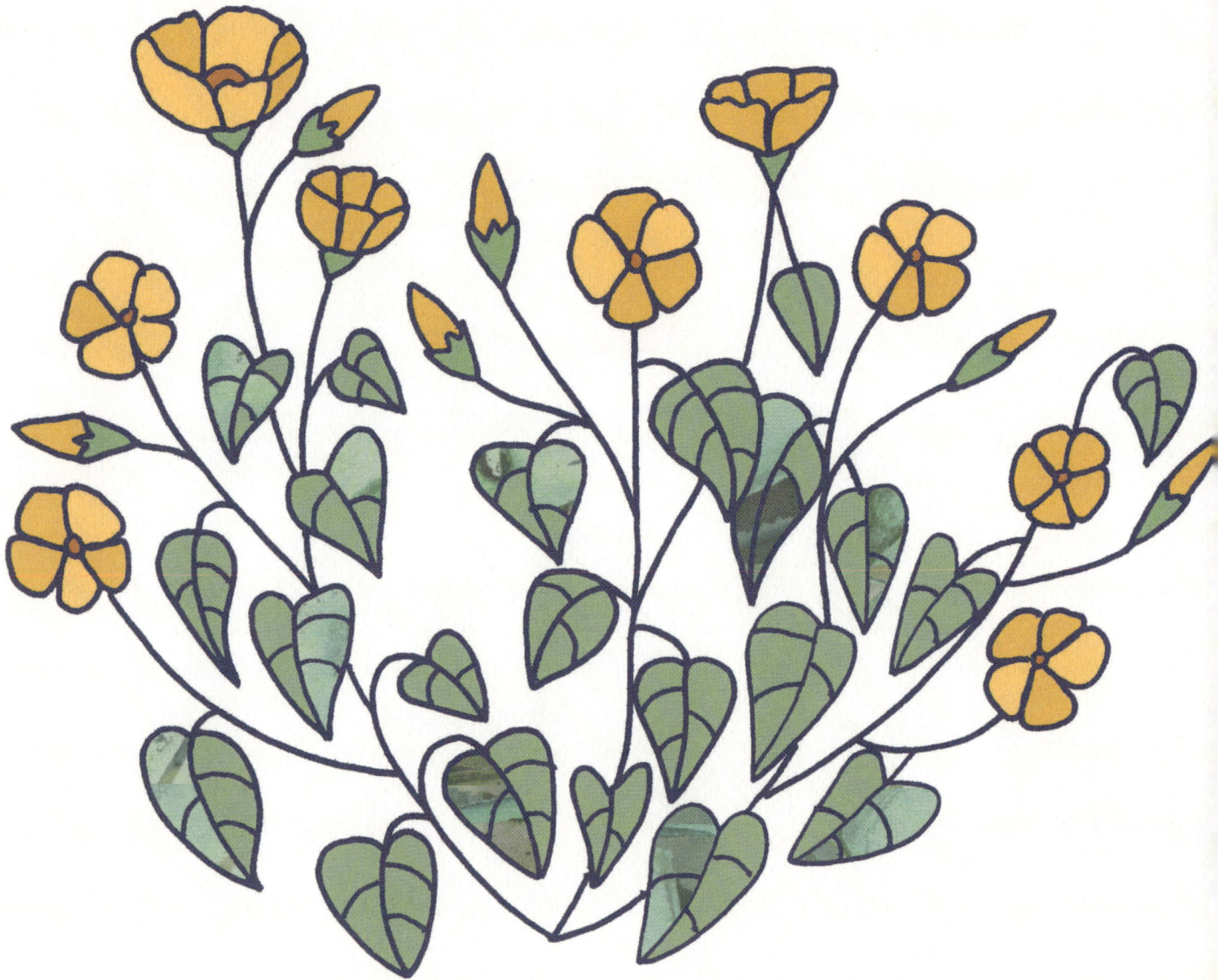

Palmer's Indian Mallow

Abutilon palmeri

Appearance: This rare, fast-growing desert wildflower shrub can grow up to 4 feet (1.2 m) tall with heart-shaped, silvery-green leaves. It has striking golden-yellow, cup-shaped flowers about 1 inch (2.5 cm) in diameter that tend to bloom almost year-round. Its seeds are formed in little clusters and tend to spread easily. Definitely an exceptional addition to any native garden.

Habitat: The Sonoran Desert and into Southern California on dry, rocky slopes in full sun between 1,800 and 2,400 feet (549 and 732 m) elevation.

Blooming season: Possible year-round.

Lifespan: Can live up to twenty years.

Environmental role: This beauty thrives with minimal water, helping to maintain vegetation and ground cover in the desert. Its deep root systems help stabilize dry, rocky slopes. It is exceptionally important for pollinators since it has a long blooming season.

Foraging: There is not much known about the historical uses of Palmer's Indian mallow specifically but it is closely related to globemallow so it can be used in many similar ways. Its leaves and flowers can be steeped into a tea to treat coughs and help hydrate. They can also be made into a poultice to treat infectious wounds. Palmer's Indian mallow is rare in the wild, so only forage if you are growing this in your garden, otherwise substitute for globemallow.

Plant friends: Globemallow and desert-rose mallow.

Purple Three-awn Grass

Aristida purpurea

Appearance: This widespread, native grass can grow up to 3 feet (91 cm) tall and 2 feet (61 cm) wide and has light-green, erect leaf blades. Three long bristles occur at each flower and the seed heads are narrow and drooping with a pretty purplish color. This grass is my favorite to find growing wild as many usually grow in patches near each other. They have a beautiful soft look to them, but they can be sharp when touched.

Habitat: Most of the Western and Midwestern United States and parts of Canada but can be found in Arizona in desert grassland, on mesas, and sandy or rocky plains in well-draining soil. Found between 1,000 and 5,000 feet (305 and 1,524 m) elevation.

Blooming season: April through October.

Lifespan: Can live up to four years with its many seeds helping it reproduce in one area.

Environmental role: Purple three-awn can thrive in arid environments and can be the first to establish itself in disturbed areas, making it ideal for desert revegetation. Its dense root systems help stabilize soil, preventing erosion. It also provides cover and nesting material for smaller desert wildlife.

Foraging: This plant has no known uses but is essential in desert grasslands to maintain a healthy ecosystem.

Plant friends: Arizona three-awn, sixweeks three-awn, and Parish's three-awn.

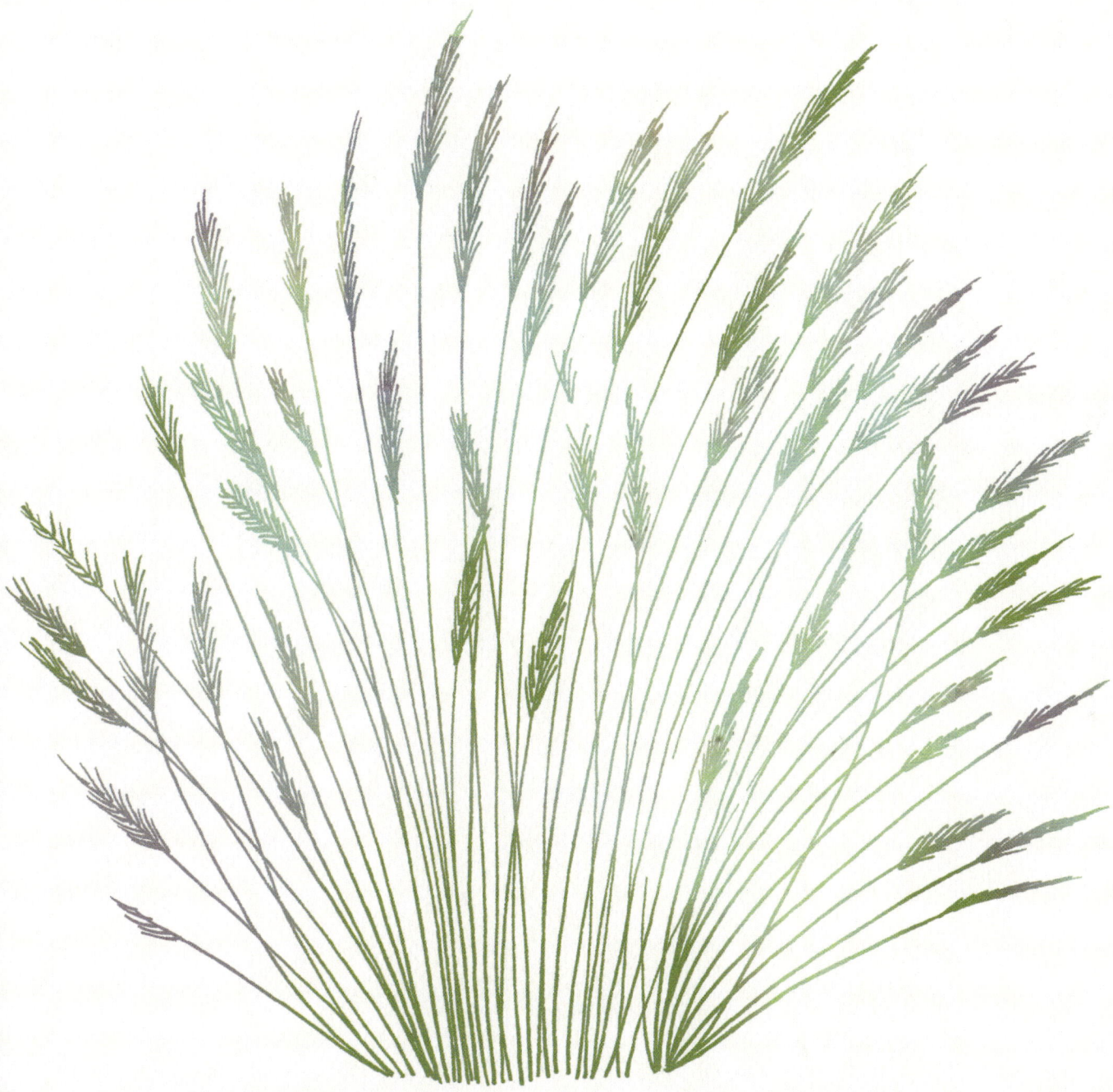

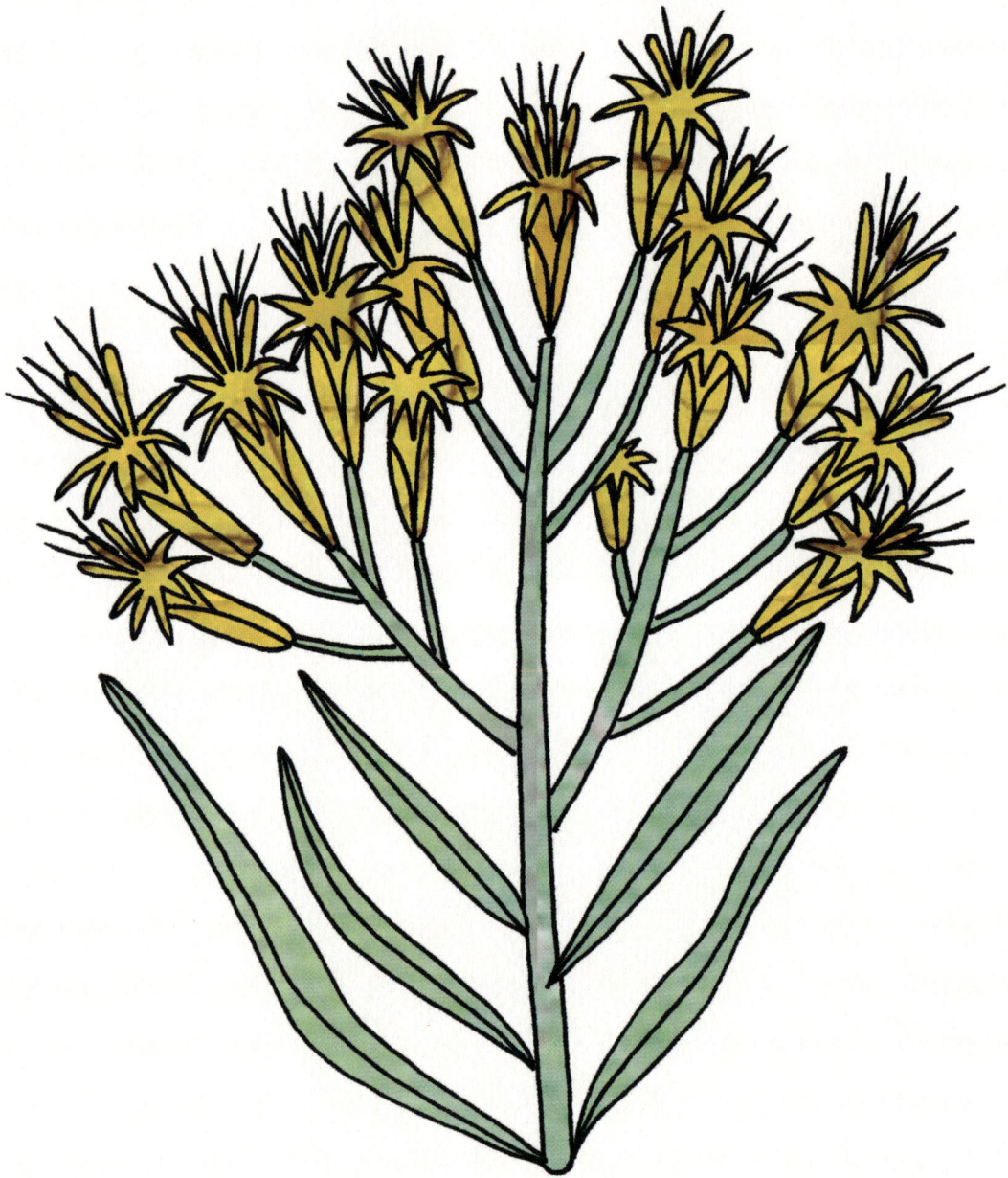

Rubber Rabbitbrush

Ericameria nauseosa

Appearance: This autumn desert beauty is an erect, slender shrub that can grow up to 8 feet (2.4 m) tall, but is often found much shorter. The flexible branches are covered with feltlike hairs with very narrow light-green to silver leaves. The ends of the stems also have small, narrow, light-green to silver leaves and small, tubular, yellow flowers that grow in clusters. They put on a real show when in full bloom and are even attractive when they start to dry out in wintertime.

Habitat: The Western United States, Western Canada and Northern Mexico in dry open plains, grassland, valleys, or open woodland between 3,000 and 9,000 feet (914 and 2,743 m) elevation.

Blooming season: August through October.

Lifespan: Can live up to twenty years.

Environmental role: These bountiful plants provide a significant nectar source for native pollinators while their foliage provides cover for small animals. Rubber rabbitbrush also serves as a food source for desert wildlife like deer. It grows quickly and can survive dry conditions which makes it excellent when revegetating challenging or degraded areas. It has also been used in a variety of ways by Indigenous peoples for thousands of years to treat a variety of ailments, for basket weaving, and for dyeing fabrics.

Foraging: This plant is widespread and common in the desert and perfect for foraging. I like to forage this plant for autumn floral arrangements because it holds its integrity when dried. A tea can be made from its flowers and leaves to relieve pain and swelling in joints and to treat diarrhea, colds, and sores. Its yellow flowers can be used to create a dye to color natural fibers—this is something I would love to try.

Plant friends: Narrowleaf goldenbush and turpentine bush.

Santa Catalina Indian Paintbrush

Castilleja tenuiflora

Appearance: This vibrant high desert wildflower stands erect up to 2 feet (61 cm) tall. The stems are hairy and green with long green leaves that are lined with purple edges and covered in white hairs. The true beauty of Santa Catalina Indian paintbrush are the many bright-red, tube-shaped flowers at the top of the stem about 1.5 inches (3.8 cm) long. From inside the red, beak-like flowers pop long, thin, tonguelike yellowish-green stigmas. The flowers turn into egg-shaped seed capsules. The ends of the flowers are reminiscent of paintbrushes, thus its name, and stand out among the rocky slopes they usually grow on.

Habitat: Arizona and New Mexico in woodlands, rocky slopes, ledges, and bedrock between 4,000 and 6,000 feet (1,219 and 1,829 m) elevation.

Blooming season: March through September.

Lifespan: This is a biennial plant, meaning it produces leaves the first year, then blooms and turns to seed the second year.

Environmental role: This wildflower is semiparasitic, meaning it draws nutrients through its interconnected root system with nearby plants so is very dependent on suitable host plants, and susceptible to human disturbance. The showy flowers of the Santa Catalina Indian paintbrush are very attractive to hummingbirds, offering them a nectar source.

Foraging: This plant is rare and shouldn't be foraged, but all Indian paintbrush variations can be used to heal skin issues like wounds, rashes, and have even been proven to shrink cancerous tumors. The flowers of Indian paintbrush can be eaten fresh or cooked, have a slightly sweet taste, and are high in vitamins and help boost the immune system.

Plant friends: Exserted Indian paintbrush, wholeleaf Indian paintbrush and Kaibab Indian paintbrush.

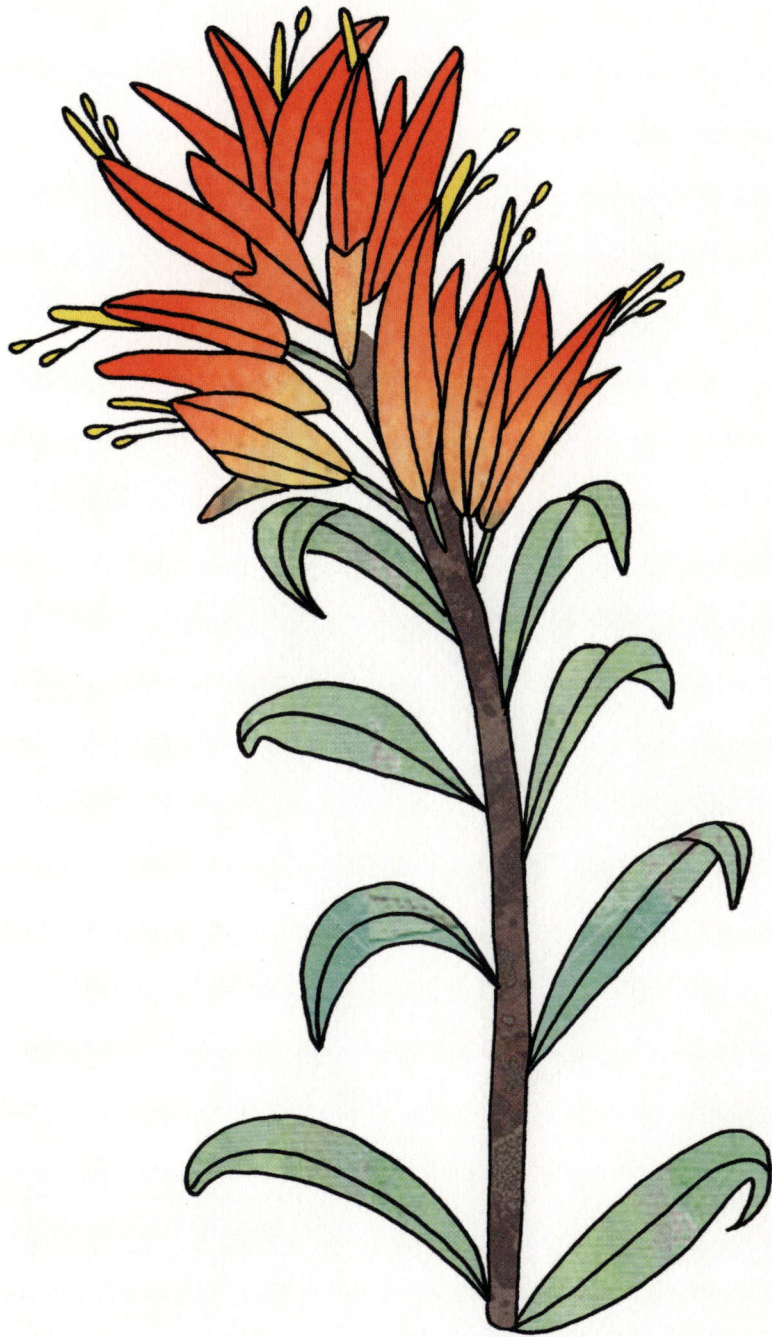

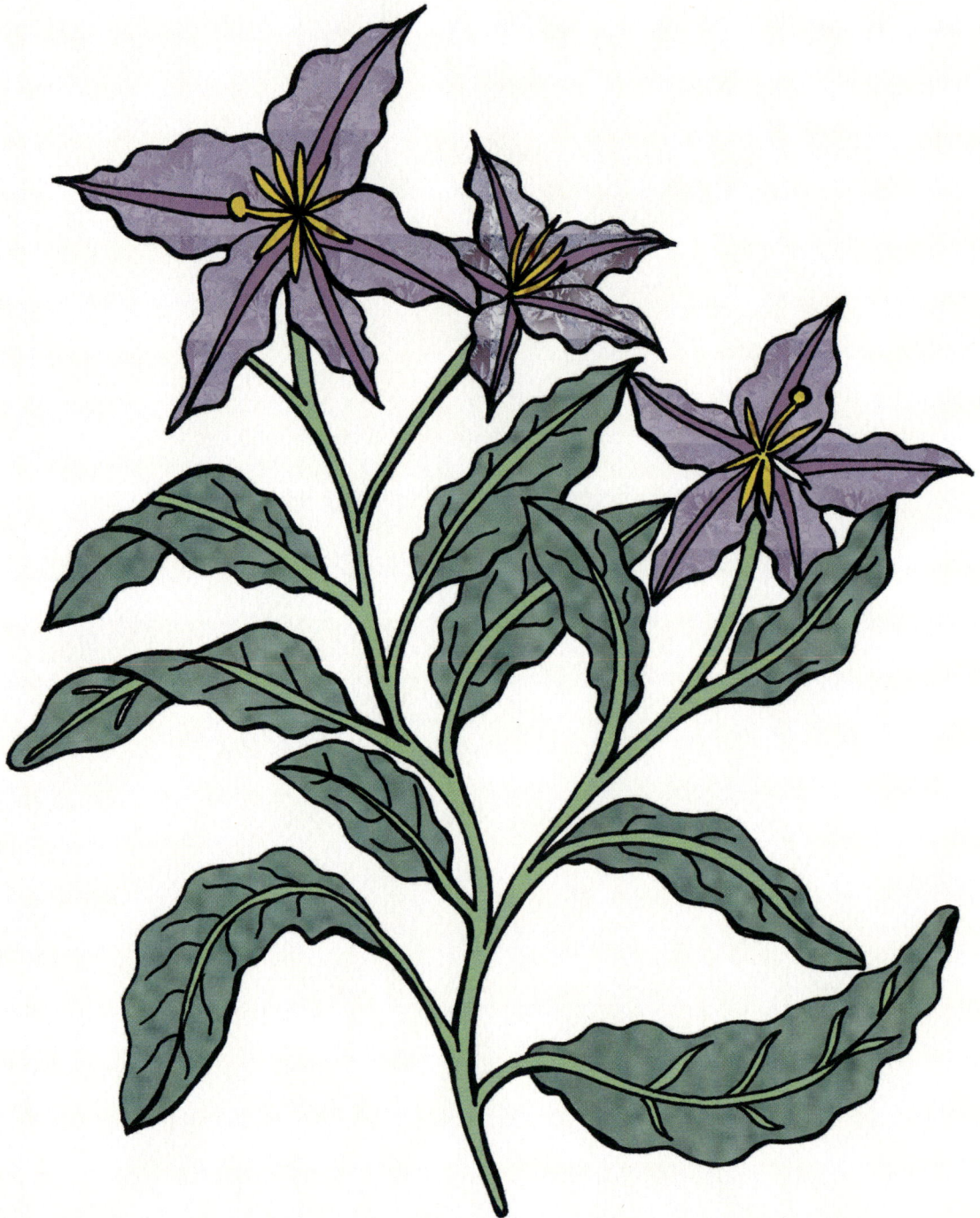

Silverleaf Nightshade

Solanum elaeagnifolium

Appearance: Silverleaf nightshade is otherworldly looking with its silvery, hairy body that can grow up to 3 feet (91 cm) tall and prominent leaves that have wavy edges about 2 to 4 inches (5 to 10 cm) long. Their five-petal blossoms are violet with a unique star shape and a bright-yellow stamen in the middle. The flowers tend to droop to one side instead of facing upward and are visually striking against their silvery bodies. They produce (probably poisonous) yellow fruits that look like small tomatoes and that can remain on the plant for many months. They usually grow close together in groups of many plants and are a delight to find!

Habitat: Much of the Southern and Western United States and Northern Mexico in prairies, fields, meadows, and pastures from sea level up to 5,500 feet (1,676 m) elevation. I see them often under and near mesquite trees.

Blooming season: May through October.

Lifespan: Can live longer than two years (perennial).

Environmental role: Many plants in the nightshade family can be toxic, and this plant is no exception. It is toxic to animals and spreads easily in disturbed areas, which gives it a bad reputation among humans. I believe any native plant has a purpose in the ecosystem and should be left alone, especially a hardy desert survivor like this one. The flowers are a great source of pollen and nectar for pollinators and it can give life to areas that other plants would not be able to grow in.

Foraging: All parts of this plant are considered toxic but Indigenous peoples applied the chewed root to snake bites to remove the venom and used the crushed berries to curdle milk. This plant should be studied more for its benefits.

Plant friends: Other nightshades like sacred datura and purple nightshade.

Southern Cattail

Typha domingensis

Appearance: These tall stalks grow up to 12 feet (4 m) high in standing freshwater in dense stands or thickets and often look like giant grass because of their long, bladelike green leaves. Their unique, petal-less flowers grow on the very tip of the spikelike stalk: the yellowish male flowers grow in a clustered, tapered cone shape above the recognizable, velvety, brown female flowers, that resemble hot dogs. The female flowers will dry and turn to fluffy, cream-colored seeds that are dispersed by wind or water. In autumn and winter, the seeds fall away from the stalk in clumps and spread all over the surrounding area.

Habitat: These tall aquatic plants are found in marshy riparian areas throughout much of the United States, generally below 7,000 feet (2,134 m) elevation.

Blooming season: March through August, but I placed these in this Autumn section because of their magical seed dispersal in autumn.

Lifespan: Perennial, though their exact lifespan is uncertain.

Environmental role: Cattails play a crucial role in aquatic environments. They reduce harmful bacteria and absorb heavy metals in the water and soil, creating a cleaner ecosystem. The clusters of stalks prevent erosion along shorelines and slow water movement which creates a calm and safe environment for wildlife to thrive in. They provide nesting material and sites for birds, and food for small mammals. Indigenous peoples used all parts of this plant, for food and weaving material.

Foraging: All parts of the southern cattail are edible. Catttails are rich in potassium, protein, amino acids, and vitamin C. The young shoots can be eaten raw or cooked in the springtime. The young flower stalks can be boiled or steamed like corn. Cattail pollen can be gathered and used like flour. Their strong leaves can be dried and used to weave baskets, mats, and more. Dried stalks make great floral arrangements. Only forage in places where there are dense areas of many cattails growing together, avoiding new populations.

Plant friends: Broadleaf cattail.

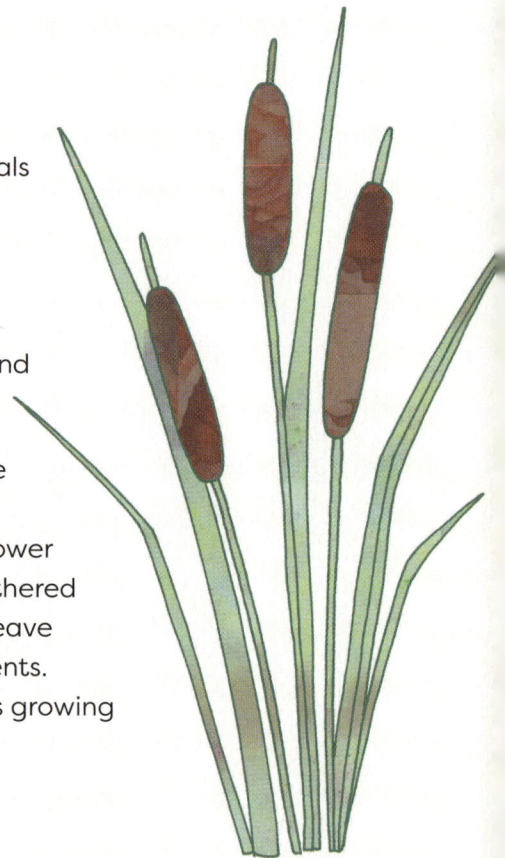

Autumn Dried Floral Arrangement

Forage and arrange cattail stalks as described below for a striking display in the late summer and early autumn—though they look beautiful for years.

MATERIALS

- Cattails (see instructions)
- Pruning shears
- Large, tall vase or decorative bucket
- Dried mesquite branches (optional)
- Recycled foam, sized to fit your vase or decorative bucket (optional)

INSTRUCTIONS

1. Find a dense thicket of cattails (in riparian areas) and approach ones along the shoreline that are easily accessible without wading into the water.

2. Using pruning shears, collect 6 to 9 stalks depending on how large an arrangement you desire: snip the stalk near the waterline for a very tall arrangement or about halfway up the stalk for a large but shorter arrangement.

3. Arrange the stalks in a tall vase or decorative bucket. You can leave the cattails by themselves for a festive look or add some thin, tall, dried mesquite branches for a more dramatic look.

4. Place the arrangement on a short table next to a wall (the wall gives them more stability when standing). Alternatively, place a piece of recycled foam in the bottom of the vase or vessel to secure each stalk into a specific place.

Wild Sunflower

Helianthus annuus

Appearance: These popular wildflowers are an autumn staple in the desert, lining roadways and arroyos with their showy, sunlike flowers. They can grow up to 9 feet (2.7 m) tall, erect with many branching flowers at the top of one plant. The bright-green stems and leaves are covered in short, coarse hairs. Their leaves are large, wide and heart shaped, growing up to 1 foot (30.5 cm) long. They are well known for their flower heads that can grow up to 5 inches (13 cm) across with a large, round, maroon disc in the middle surrounded by long, thin, bright-yellow petals. Wild sunflowers are one of my favorite autumn flowers to run into while out foraging.

Habitat: Throughout North America between 100 and 7,000 feet (30 and 2,134 m) elevation in riparian communities, grasslands, disturbed areas, roadsides, and more.

Blooming season: June through October.

Lifespan: Annual.

Environmental role: We all know sunflower seeds are edible and wild sunflower seeds are an important source of food for birds and small mammals, especially because these plants produce so many seeds in late autumn and winter. Their flowers are also important for local pollinators. They are extremely helpful for detoxifying soil as they absorb heavy metals and nitrates through their roots—called phytoremediation.

Foraging: Sunflowers may seem appealing to forage for their seeds or for floral arrangements, but they do not look very pretty when dried and their seeds are best left for wildlife. Instead, I enjoy sitting and admiring them.

Plant friends: Prairie sunflower, Arizona sunflower.

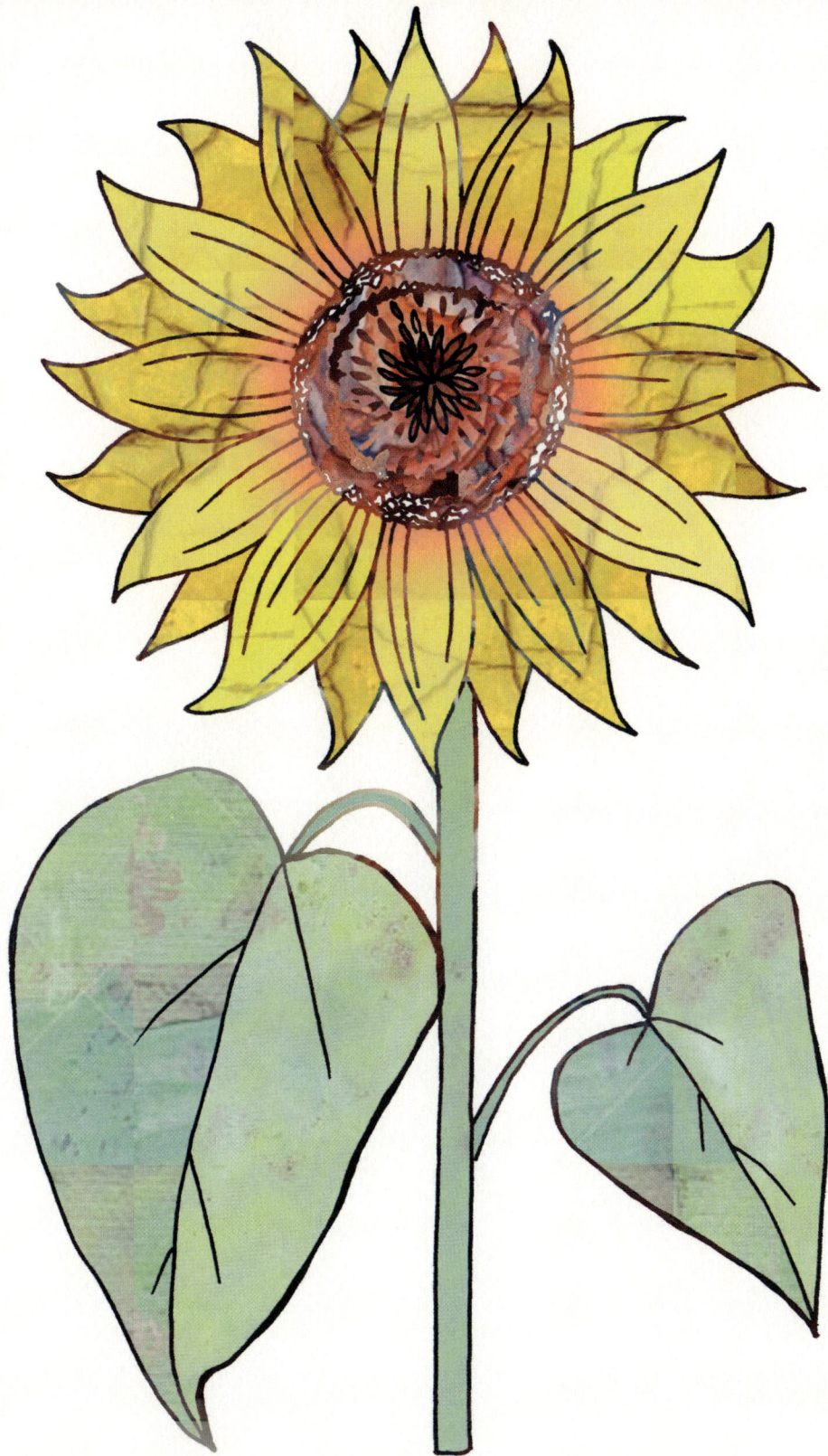

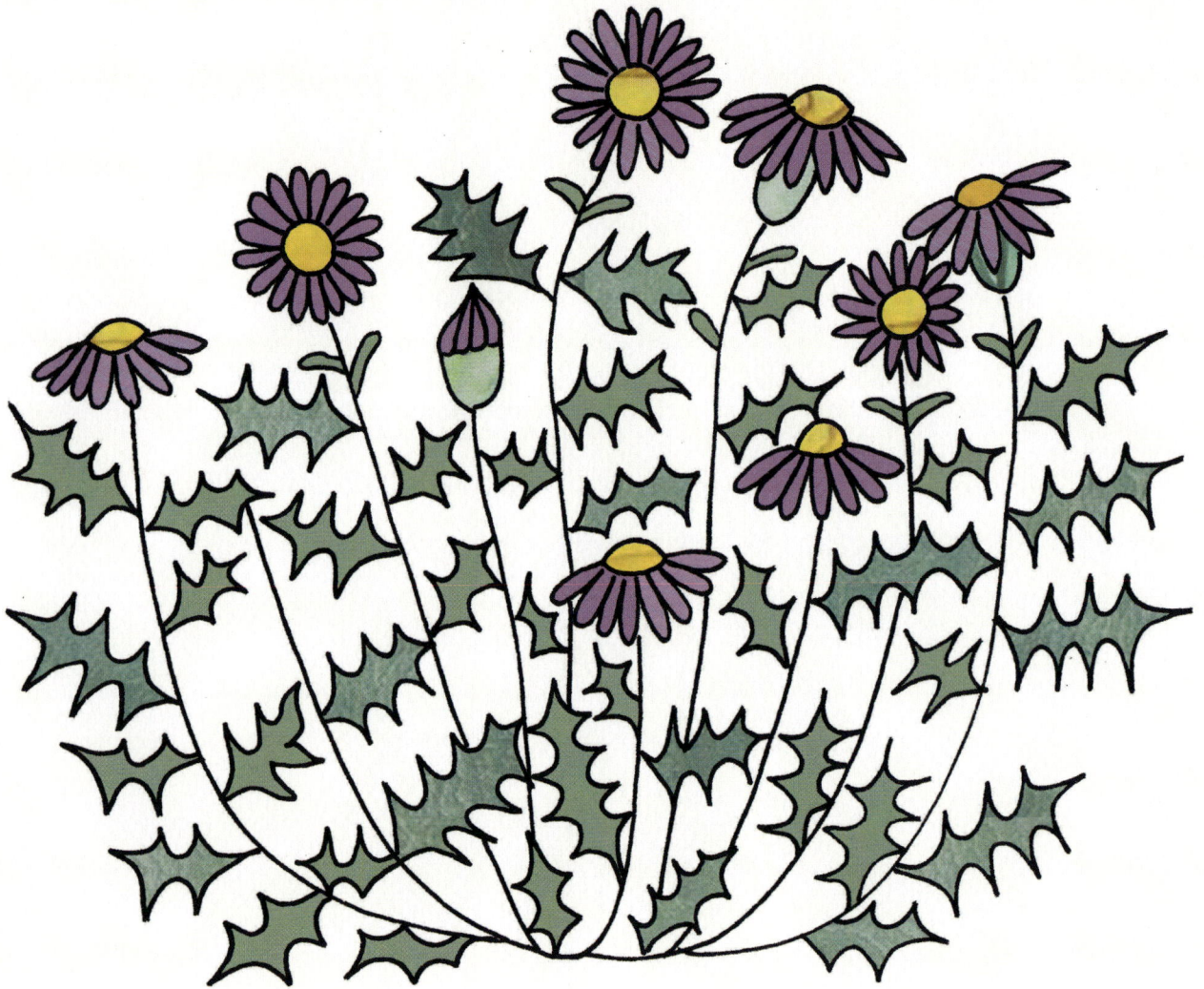

Tansyleaf Tansyaster

Machaeranthera tanacetifolia

Appearance: These little bright-purple flowers always stand out among the greens and browns of the Sonoran Desert. This plant has numerous erect green stems covered in sticky, fine hairs and can grow up to 2 feet (61 cm) tall. It has many fernlike, dissected leaves that are also hairy with tiny spines. It has small, 1 inch (2.5 cm) wide, daisylike flowers composed of a bright yellow disc surrounded by thin lavender petals. One plant can grow many delicate flowers at the ends of the multibranched stems.

Habitat: Central and Southwestern United States, Northern Mexico and Alberta, Canada, in a wide range of drier habitats like the Rocky Mountains, Great Plains, desert grasslands, chaparral communities, and woodlands between 2,500 and 8,000 feet (762 and 2,438 m) elevation.

Blooming season: April through October.

Lifespan: Because Tansyleaf tansyaster can grow in a variety of habitats, it can be either a biennial plant (living up to two years to complete its full life cycle) or perennial (living longer than two years).

Environmental role: This flower attracts a wide range of pollinators with its nectar-rich flowers, so supports biodiversity, especially in drier areas where flowers may be scarce. Its seeds are also an important food source for small mammals and birds. It helps prevent soil erosion with its root system and can thrive in a large range of environments, making it highly adaptable. Native peoples like the Hopi, Navajo, and Ramah have used this plant medicinally.

Foraging: This plant can be used medicinally, though it has not been studied. It can be made into a tea to treat stomachaches or as a stimulant. Its roots can be used as a respiratory aid. Proceed with caution and common sense if using this plant medicinally.

Plant friends: Mesa tansyaster and arid tansyaster.

Winter

The Dormant Season

December through February

The seasons change slowly in the desert. We look to the subtleties like the chill in the evening breeze and the cold dew that rests on the ground in the early mornings. We cherish our few winter months, both indoors and out. We spend our time outdoors being warmed by the sun. Inside, we sip tea and cuddle around the piñon pine log burning in the chiminea: another reminder of the season. Many of us head to our sky islands to feel the winter nostalgia that so many of us see in storybooks. There the white snow blankets the mountain peaks and dresses the high desert trees.

The vanilla scent of the tall ponderosa pine fills the air. Our conifers are fragrant, strong, and steadfast, showing us the strength we seek. We spend time together with loved ones and celebrate life. Winter is a time to care for each other, enjoy the year's harvest, sow our seeds for spring, relax, and wait for the next season to sprout.

Winter is a dormant time for the Sonoran Desert. The wildflowers of spring and the greenery of summer are distant memories as we step into the cold winter months. The temperatures in the valleys rarely go below freezing but the mountains at higher elevations will stay below freezing and will see snow regularly. Very rarely will winter snow stay on the ground in the desert biomes, but it is always a nice little gift to see the tall saguaros covered in it. The desert is usually dry during this season, save for an occasional soft rain. I pray for rain at this time of year because plentiful winter rain means a bountiful spring. Being an Arizona native, I find that winter is harsh to me. I prefer the heat and could never survive a colder environment. Most other people are happy to have a respite from the heat, and snowbirds (people who live here part-time in the cooler months) fill the desert cities as they look to get away from colder climates. However, temperatures start to increase in February as winter slowly makes way for spring and we can start to see some of the spring wildflowers sprouting.

As nature slows down and most everything stops growing in the winter, the desert displays its classic landscape look: dry, brown, with speckles of cactus on the horizon. Here, I will be going over some of the mainstays of the Sonoran Desert as they are the only constants throughout every season, and are easily noticeable in the winter due to the lack of other seasonal flora.

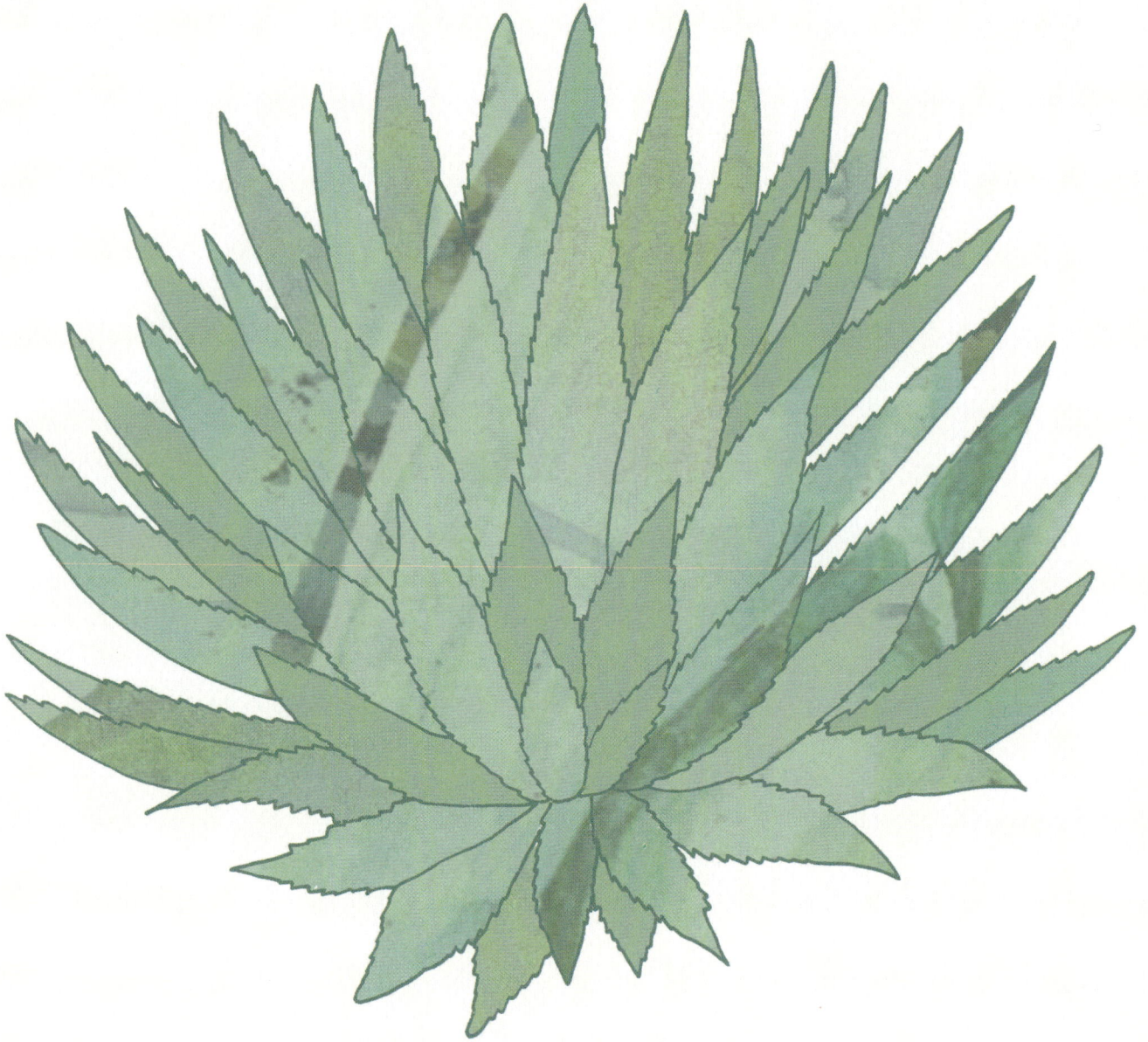

Arizona Agave

Agave x arizonica

Appearance: This hybrid between *Agave chrysantha* and *Agave tourneyana v. bella* is a rare gem described, by the few that have seen it, as one of the most beautiful agaves in Arizona. It has distinct bright-green, spiked leaves with dark brown edges. It is small, usually a single rosette not usually growing over 1 foot (30.5 cm) tall and a little over 1 foot (30.5 cm) across. Like most agaves, its leaves have sharp spines on their tips and along their sides. It has a tall, thin, woody stalk that produces yellow, jar-shaped flowers.

Habitat: Arizona agave is endemic to a very small area of the state, on steep, rocky granite hills or on hilltops among chaparral- and juniper-dominated grasslands. Has been documented in the Tonto National Forest at an elevation around 3,000 feet (914 m).

Blooming season: March through July.

Lifespan: Fifteen to twenty years.

Environmental role: This rare agave offers similar environmental and sociological benefits to other agaves. It helps prevent soil erosion, is a great survivor, and can easily propagate itself through pups (clones of itself growing near the origin plant). The flowers offer food to pollinators and humans can use this plant in a variety of ways (although it is tough to work with).

Threats: Because this plant is a hybrid, it is rare and groups like the Desert Botanical Garden in Phoenix, Arizona, are making efforts to conserve it.

Foraging: This plant is rare and should not be foraged.

Plant friends: *Agave chrysantha* and *Agave tourneyana v. bella* are great friends of this plant as they hybridized together to create Arizona agave!

Arrowweed

Pluchea sericea

Appearance: A tall, thin, bushy shrub with grayish-green linear, fuzzy leaves. The tubular flower heads grow in clusters and range from pink to fuchsia (almost looking like tiny thistles). It forms a dense thicket with many other plants growing around it.

Habitat: Grows wild in the Southwestern United States and Northern Mexico, but primarily found in Arizona and Southern California. Found in moist riparian desert areas like washes, rivers, stream banks, and springs. I have personally found it along the banks of the Santa Cruz River.

Blooming season: January through July.

Lifespan: Uncertain, but I would estimate three to eight years based on my experience.

Environmental role: This thick plant gives cover for wildlife as they approach water sources. Because it grows on the banks of water sources, it helps prevent soil erosion with its root system. Its seeds are a food source and flowers a nectar source for wildlife. Arrowweed stems have been used by many Southwestern Indigenous peoples to make arrow shafts and craft thatching for shelters. It is also medicinal, and its roots have been used as an eyewash and as a gastrointestinal aid for issues like diarrhea.

Foraging: Arrowweed has culinary as well as medicinal functions; the roots can be roasted and consumed. Arrowweed has a distinct scent: slightly sweet with notes of camphor. I have considered creating a natural perfume from this plant but haven't yet experimented with it. This plant grows vivaciously near water sources and its full range of benefits have yet to be explored by modern science.

Plant friends: Arrowweed is closely related to salt marsh fleabane, which often grows near other riparian desert plants.

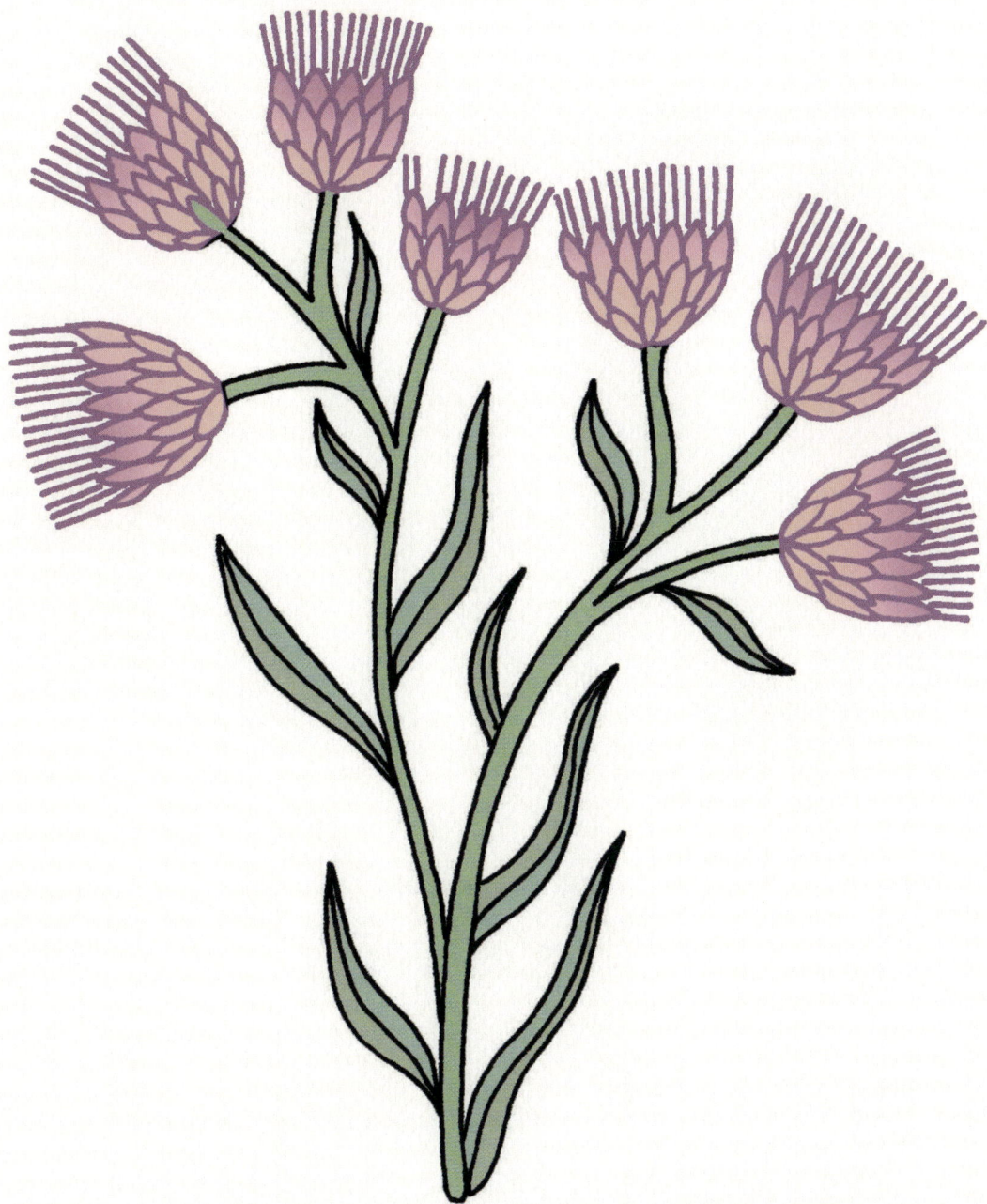

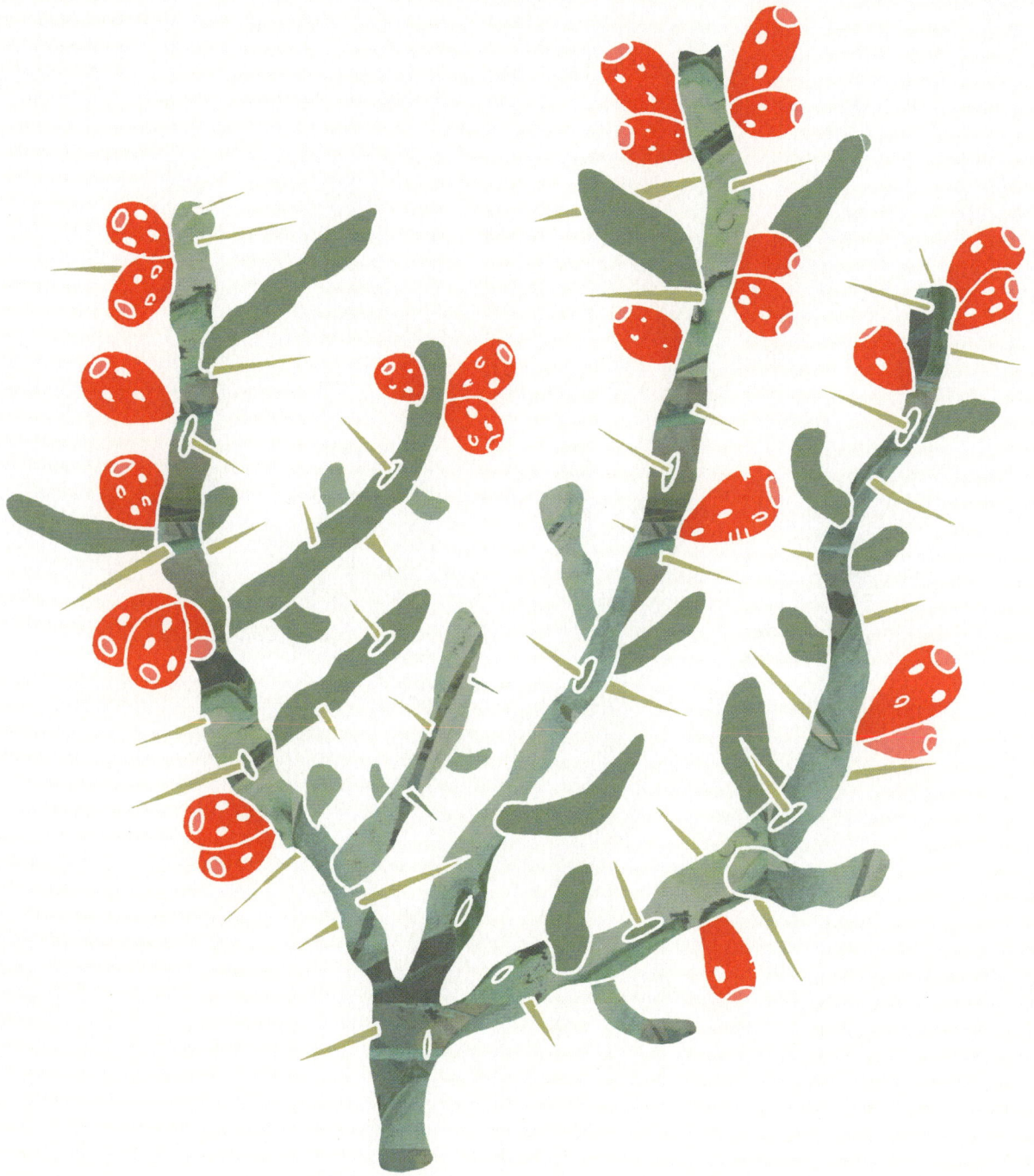

Christmas Cholla

Cylindropuntia leptocaulis

Appearance: This thin, upright desert cactus is unsuspecting as it can blend into the spiny landscape around it—until its bright-red fruits show themselves in autumn and winter, giving it its name. It can grow up to 5 feet (1.5 m) tall and is made up of long, thin, cylindrical joints covered in small spines and glochids. Its new growth is a dark-green color but with age it turns a scaly pale brown. It produces small, beautiful, yellowish-green flowers in the spring which then turn to fleshy, barrel-shaped fruits that start green and slowly ripen to a bright-red color.

Habitat: Found in the Sonoran and Chihuahuan Deserts and Northern Mexico between 1,000 and 5,000 feet (305 and 1,524 m) elevation in valleys, desert washes, mesas, and flatlands.

Blooming season: April through August but it is more known for its ripe fruits in the winter.

Lifespan: Can live up to fifteen years.

Environmental role: Christmas cholla provides shelter for small desert wildlife and its roots help stabilize the soil. Cacti like this cholla play a crucial role in the desert's water cycle because they absorb and store water for long periods of time. Their fruits are an important food source for wildlife and Indigenous peoples.

Foraging: Though small, the raw, ripe fruits of this cholla are actually pretty tasty compared to other cholla. I like to pull one off using two sticks and use rocks to rub the glochids (tiny spines) off of the fruit to eat while on the trail. I am sure there are plenty of ways to make use of this fruit, but I tend to only eat a few at a time. The flavor varies from plant to plant and with differing levels of ripeness.

Plant friends: Teddy bear cholla and staghorn cholla.

Chuparosa

Justicia californica

Appearance: Chuparosa is a rare succulent-like shrub with green, twiggy stems that can grow up to 6 feet (1.8 m) tall and nearly twice as wide. It has small, bright-green, oval leaves that drop off the plant in the hotter summer months. These plants are most known for their plentiful, bright-red (sometimes reddish-orange), funnel-shaped flowers that bloom at the ends of the stems. I call flowers like these hummingbird trumpets because they are perfectly shaped for tiny, long beaks to reach the nectar inside.

Habitat: Only in Arizona and California between 1,000 and 4,000 feet (305 and 1,219 m) elevation in desert washes and rocky slopes.

Blooming season: Can be found throughout the year (except summer), but the most plentiful blooms occur during winter and early spring.

Lifespan: At least three years, though most likely much longer—the exact lifespan is uncertain.

Environmental role: This tolerant plant can survive in poor soil and extreme heat, making it a wonderful desert plant. Chuparosa is a hummingbird and pollinator haven because it yields so many flowers on one plant and blooms often, including in the winter when so many other desert plants are dormant. I have personally witnessed one bush swarming with about fifteen different species of pollinator. Many happy pollinators mean a balanced and healthy ecosystem. Indigenous and Hispanic peoples have also used chuparosa as a source of food and medicine for thousands of years.

Foraging: Chuparosa, though rare, has a multitude of uses. The flowers are often consumed raw and in salads and are known to contain essential amino acids and other health benefits. Chuparosa has long been used to treat respiratory conditions, skin irritations, and rheumatism and can also be used in dyeing textiles. Since chuparosa is hard to find in the wild, consider planting in your home garden to benefit from its wide range of uses.

Plant friends: Thurber's desert honeysuckle and Arizona foldwing.

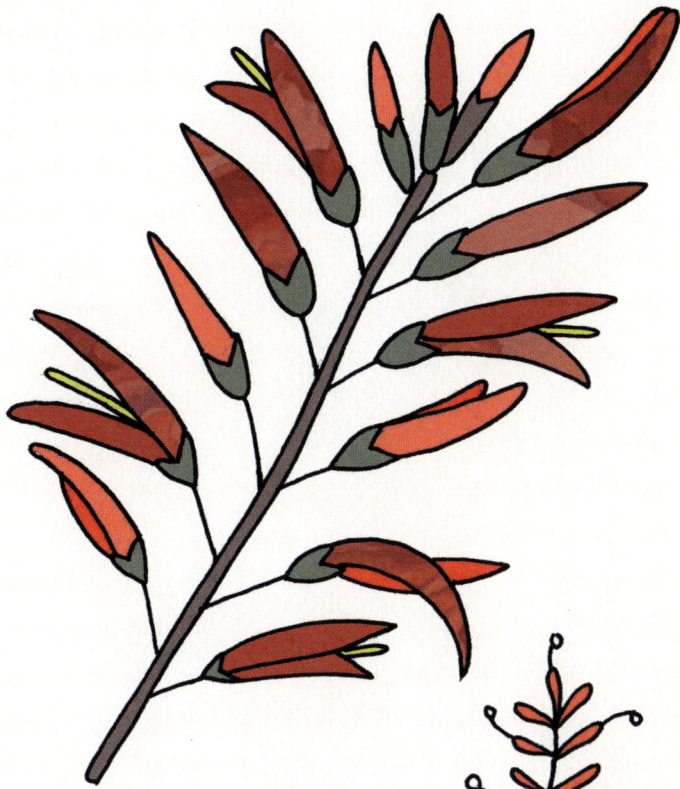

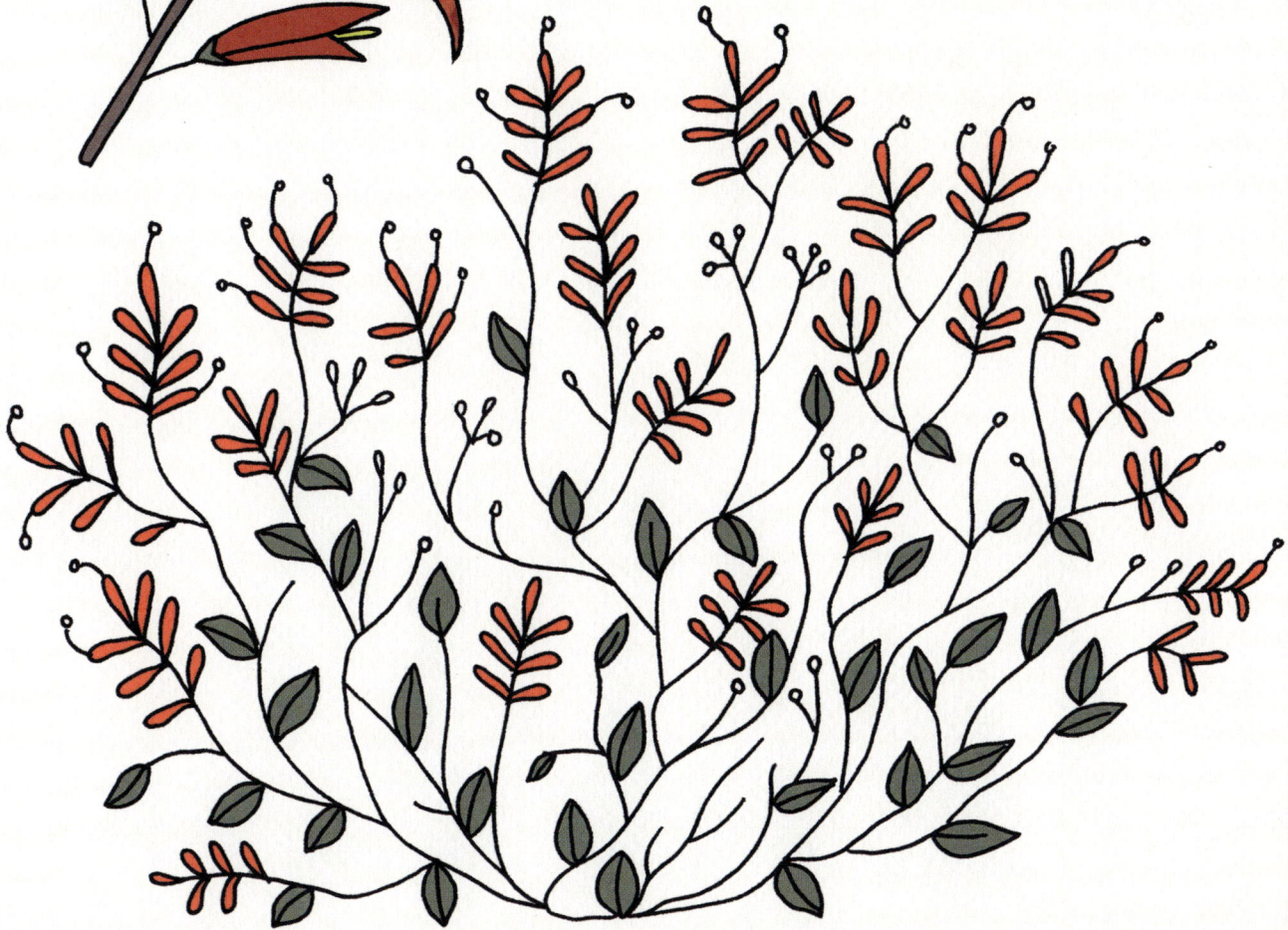

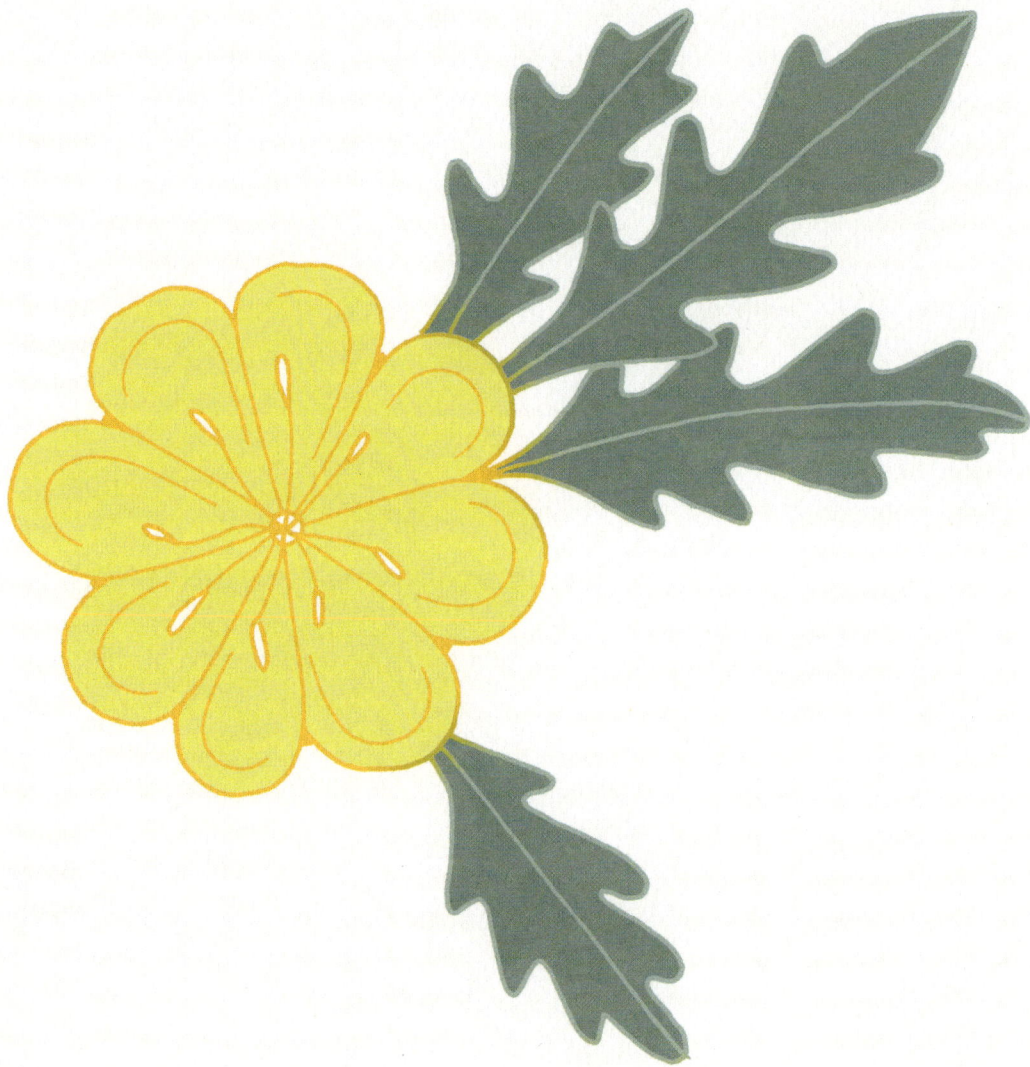

Desert Evening Primrose

Oenothera primiveris

Appearance: This gorgeous flower is one of my favorite night-blooming desert plants. Desert evening primrose is a small plant that grows in clumps, low to the ground, only reaching up to 1 foot (30.5 cm) tall. It has long, green leaves with undulating clefts on the edges that spread into a prostrate (stretched out on the ground) rosette with no long stems. The canary-yellow flowers have four petals and can grow up to 2 inches (5 cm) across. The flowers fade to orange or red as the flower ages.

Habitat: Found in the Southwestern United States and Northwestern Mexico below 4,500 feet (1,372 m) elevation in dry open deserts, sandy dunes, and arroyos (only after adequate winter rainfall).

Blooming season: February through June.

Lifespan: Annual.

Environmental role: This plant can be the first to grow in disturbed areas, making way for longer-living plants. It attracts and is a food source for pollinators because of its large, showy flowers. It is a food source for caterpillars such as the white-lined sphinx (which eventually turns into the beautiful white-lined sphinx moth). It has been used as a dermatological aid among the Navajo.

Foraging: Evening primroses are most well known for their beneficial seed oils, even though oils aren't normally extracted from this variety. I use evening primrose oil in a face oil that clears acne—Desert Primrose Creosote Face Oil. The leaves of desert evening primrose can be eaten, similar to spinach. This plant is not super common in the Sonoran Desert so foraging should be limited but it can be grown in home gardens.

Plant friends: Mexican evening primrose and Arizona evening primrose.

Desert Mistletoe

Phoradendron californicum

Appearance: This succulent-like hemiparasitic plant grows off of the branches of desert legume trees like mesquite, palo verde, ironwood, and acacia. It has long, light green, thin, leafless stems that photosynthesize, but the roots of this plant are attached to the branches of its host tree or shrub and absorb water and nutrients through them. They produce tons of small white berries that turn a salmon color when ripe and each contain several sticky red seeds. Birds will eat these berries and drop their seeds through their fecal matter onto the branches; this is one way the desert mistletoe seeds attach themselves to the host branches. If too many desert mistletoe plants establish themselves on a host tree then the tree will die due to lack of nutrients.

Habitat: It can be found in the Sonoran and Mojave Deserts up to 4,600 feet (1,402 m) elevation anywhere its host trees grow.

Blooming season: January through March.

Lifespan: Can live up to seventy years!

Environmental role: When I first learned about desert mistletoe, years ago, I thought of it as a disease, but after observing and learning more, I realized this plant is an essential part of the desert ecosystem. It provides so much food for birds and other wildlife because it produces so many berries and lives so long. A healthy tree can disarm a newly growing desert mistletoe, so it seems the desert trees that are taken over by desert mistletoe may have been elderly or sick to start with. The plant also produces pollen and nectar for native pollinators and its dense cover provides nesting sites for birds. Many Indigenous peoples consumed the ripe berries. Their benefits seem to outweigh their detriments.

Foraging: Though many mistletoe berries are toxic, and desert mistletoe stems are toxic, the desert mistletoe berries are edible when ripe (reddish and translucent) and have a slightly sweet and tart flavor. The berries can be used in a variety of ways, cooked or eaten raw. When the berries look ripe, the best way to forage (a method used by the native Seri people) is to spread a blanket underneath the plant and use a stick to shake the berries loose. The stems can be used to create a beige-colored dye for textiles. These plants are plentiful in the Sonoran Desert but try not to harm the plant itself while foraging berries.

Plant friends: Colorado desert mistletoe.

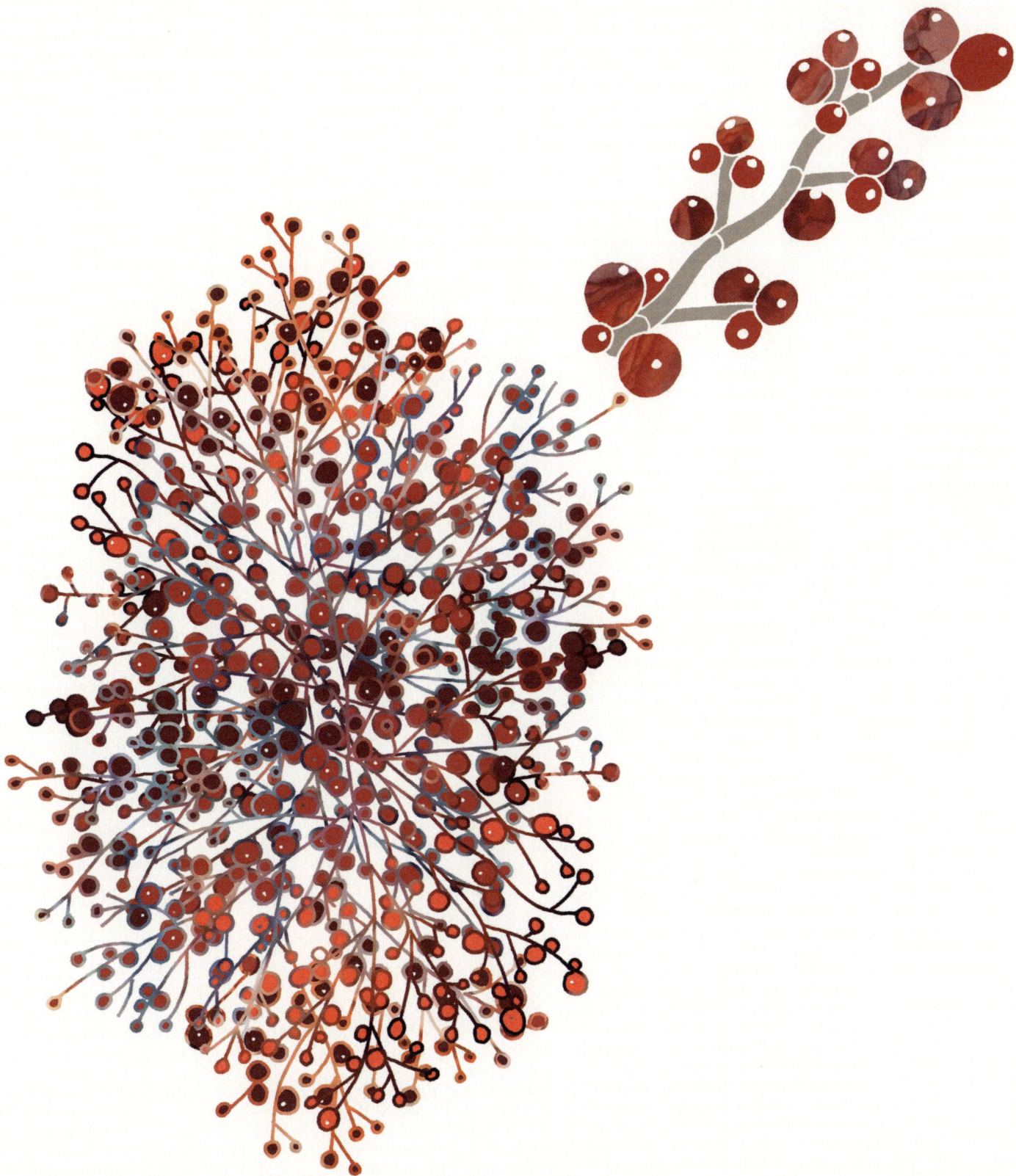

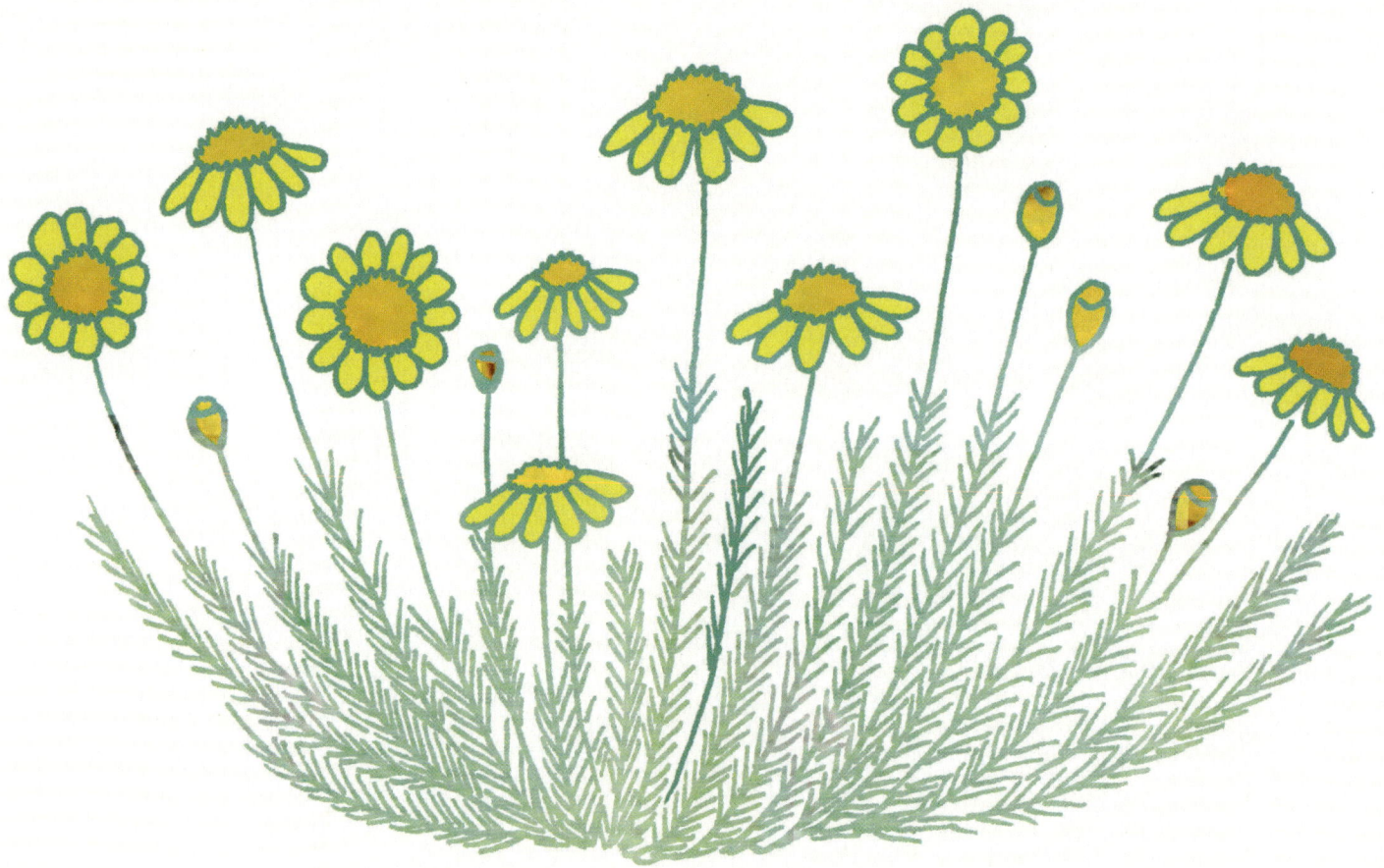

Fiveneedle Pricklyleaf

Thymophylla pentachaeta

Appearance: These small, low-growing beauties make for lovely ground cover. They grow in dense dark-green mounds with small, threadlike, cleft leaves that are spined at the tip (though not painful to touch). The entire plant can only grow up to 8 inches (20 cm) tall, usually smaller. The small, deep-yellow, daisylike flowers grow at the tip of a leafless stem and are about ½ inch (1 cm) across. I love to see these wildflowers in early winter and throughout the spring, usually growing near the safety of a prickly pear cactus or creosote bush. This plant gives off a strong camphor scent when crushed.

Habitat: Throughout the Southwestern United States and Northern Mexico between 2,400 and 4,500 feet (732 and 1,372 m) elevation in a wide range of habitats, but mostly lower and higher desert areas, mesas, and rocky or dry hillsides.

Blooming season: Year-round with adequate rainfall or water source.

Lifespan: Depending on rainfall and water sources it can live for one or more years (annual or perennial).

Environmental role: These small, showy flowers are beneficial to native bees and other pollinators because they continually bloom into multiple seasons, offering nectar when nectar might be scarce. Their seeds are a food source for small mammals and birds and the entire plant is used as cover for small wildlife.

Foraging: Used decoratively—I forage these little flowers to decorate the soap and bath bombs I create. Very cute when pressed and dried. Great for growing in gardens and yards.

Plant friends: Pricklyleaf dogweed and Sonoran pricklyleaf.

Fremont Wolfberry

Lycium fremontii

Appearance: This large, dense shrub goes mostly unnoticed among the spiny desert landscape until it blooms and fruits. Fremont wolfberry can grow up to 10 feet (3 m) tall and 8 feet (2.4 m) wide. It has long, thin, gray, hairy, intricate stems with weak spines along them. It grows thick, green, oval-shaped leaves that can fall off during drought and remerge with rainfall. Its flowers are small, tubular, and purple growing up to ½ inch (1 cm) long, with many on one plant. It is well known for its edible goji berries that are reddish orange and pea sized. One plant can produce a massive number of berries. One of my favorite desert snacks!

Habitat: Only found in Arizona and California between 300 and 4,300 feet (91 and 1,311 m) elevation along washes, slopes, and desert areas.

Blooming season: February through May and August through December.

Lifespan: The exact lifespan of this rarer plant is uncertain but other similar wolfberry plants can live up to ninety years.

Environmental role: The Fremont wolfberry bush plays an important role in the desert ecosystem. It creates cover and protection for desert wildlife and its flowers are a nectar source for desert pollinators. It is most important for the multitude of edible fruit it gives to wildlife, especially birds. Many Indigenous peoples also benefit from this powerful, nutrient-rich food source.

Foraging: These tasty desert goji berries are packed full of antioxidants and vitamin C that can boost our immune system. They also help stabilize blood sugar and improve liver function. These berries have been consumed in many different ways by the Indigenous peoples of Arizona and can be cooked, boiled, dried, and eaten raw. I like to make baked goods with these berries or dry them in the sun like raisins if I don't plan on eating them right away. I collect just enough to use for what I plan on preparing and leave the rest for the wildlife.

Plant friends: There are many types of wolfberries (Lycium) in Arizona: Berlandier's wolfberry, desert wolfberry, and Arizona desert thornbush to name a few (all of the berries are edible).

Desert Wolfberry Jam

MATERIALS

- 1 cup (340 g) foraged and rinsed ripe wolfberries
- ½ cup (120 ml) honey
- 1 tablespoon lemon juice
- 16-ounce (0.5 L) sanitized glass jar with lid, for storage

INSTRUCTIONS

1. Combine all ingredients in a small saucepan and cook over low heat (to preserve the nutrients), stirring occasionally until the berries have softened and released their juices (about 20 minutes).

2. Using a fork or small potato masher, mash the berries to a paste-like consistency.

3. Return the saucepan to low heat and simmer for about 30 to 40 minutes or until the mixture has thickened and reduced to about half its original volume.

4. Remove the saucepan from the heat and let sit until it's reached room temperature.

5. Transfer the jam to the sanitized jar and store in the refrigerator for up to 2 weeks.

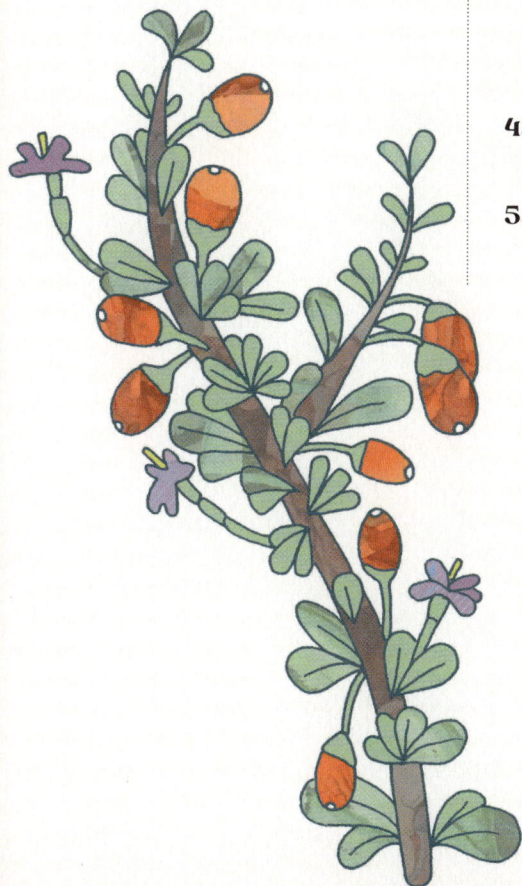

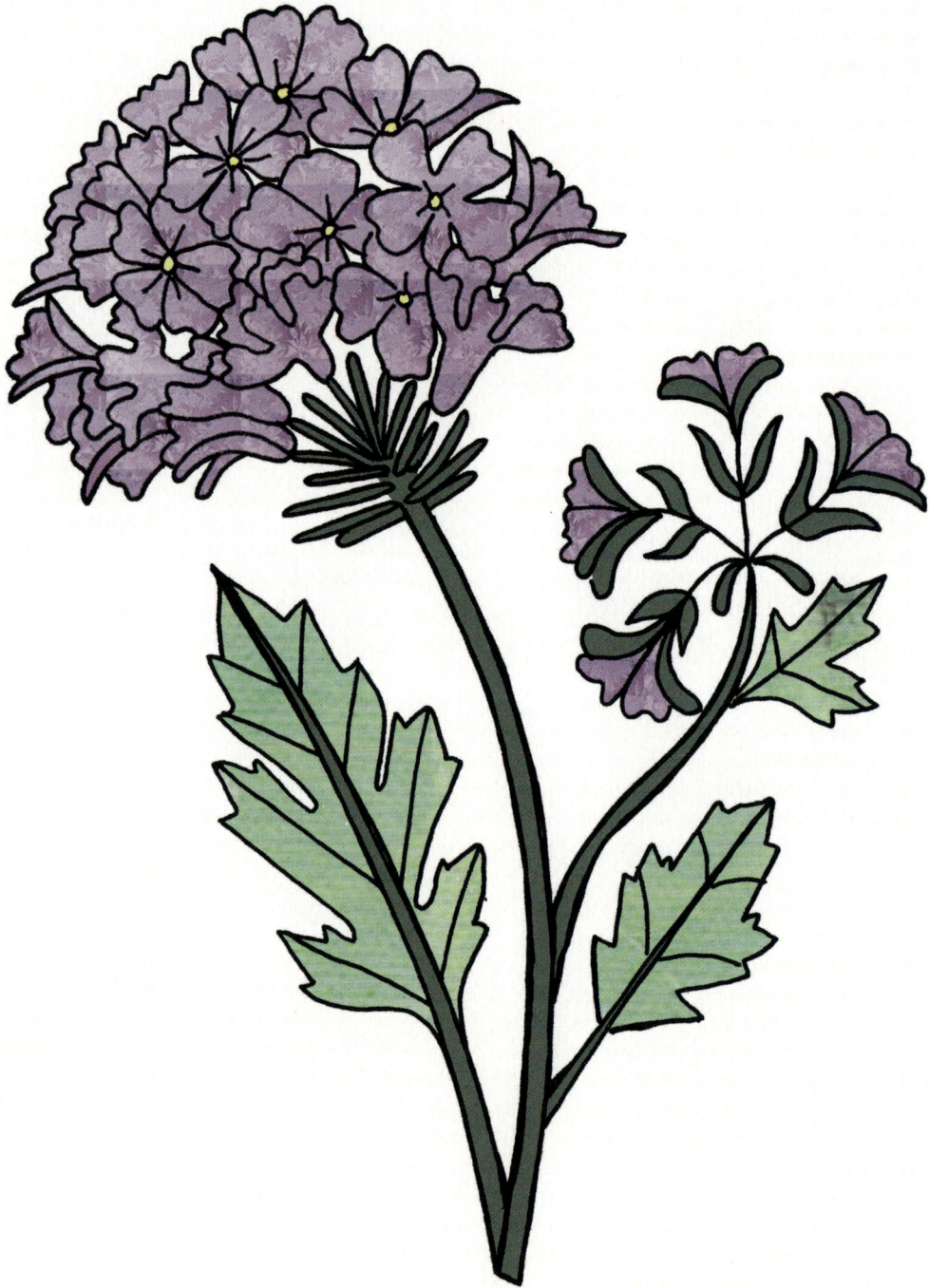

Goodding's Verbena

Glandularia gooddingii

Appearance: Goodding's verbena is a gorgeous, hairy desert wildflower. It forms a low-growing mat up to 3 feet (91 cm) wide and 1½ feet (46 cm) tall. The leaves are green and oval shaped with three major points on each leaf and a fuzzy texture, about 1 to 2 inches (2.5 to 5 cm) long. The tiny tubular flowers grow in a rounded cluster at the top of each stem with many flowers blooming on one plant. The flowers can range in color from pink, to purple, to purplish blue. They are a lovely surprise when found walking in the high desert or desert canyons.

Habitat: Found in the Southwestern United States and Mexico between 3,500 and 6,400 feet (1,067 and 1,951 m) elevation on rocky slopes, washes, mesas, and piñon forests.

Blooming season: February through April.

Lifespan: Two to three years.

Environmental role: They provide excellent ground cover, keeping the earth cooler in the warmer months. They provide food sources for desert pollinators and are very attractive in desert landscaping. They also help prevent soil erosion in sandy areas.

Foraging: This plant has no known uses but is related to verbenas so may have similar pain relieving and skin healing properties.

Plant friends: Prairie verbena and hoary vervain.

Gordon's Bladderpod

Physaria gordonii

Appearance: This early bloomer is often the first sign that spring is coming here in the Sonoran Desert, with its little yellow flowers blanketing expansive areas. It is a small, thin, erect wildflower with multiple stems on one plant and thin, green, lance-shaped leaves that can grow up to 18 inches (46 cm) tall. It grows unique small yellow flowers with four petals at the end of the stems which turn into a spherical fruit pod (thus the name bladderpod).

Habitat: Found in Southwestern and Central United States and Northern Mexico below 5,000 feet (1,524 m) elevation along dry plains, mountain slopes, and mesas.

Blooming season: February through May.

Lifespan: Annual.

Environmental role: This plant is a very vital source of forage for many desert animals like deer because it starts to grow in late winter, when much green forage is dormant. Its seeds are also consumed by birds and small mammals.

Foraging: The seeds are edible for humans but only if cooked. Foraging these small seeds would be time consuming but they have a flavor similar to peas and are rich in nutrients.

Plant friends: Fendler's bladderpod and common pepperweed.

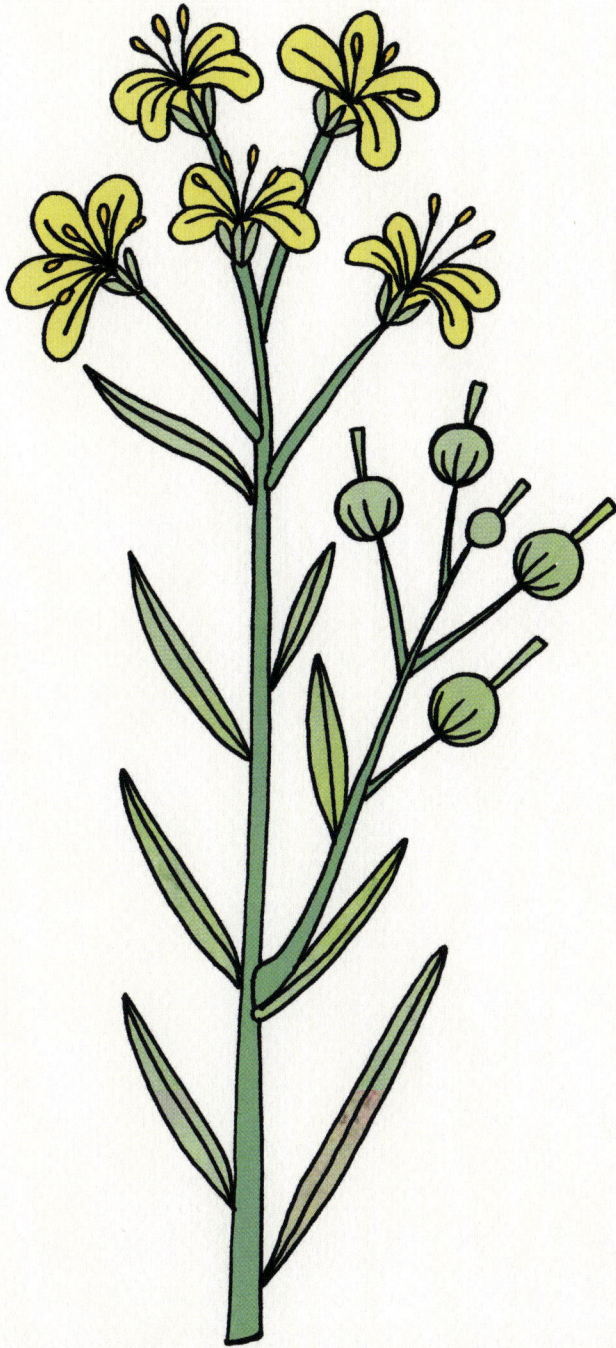

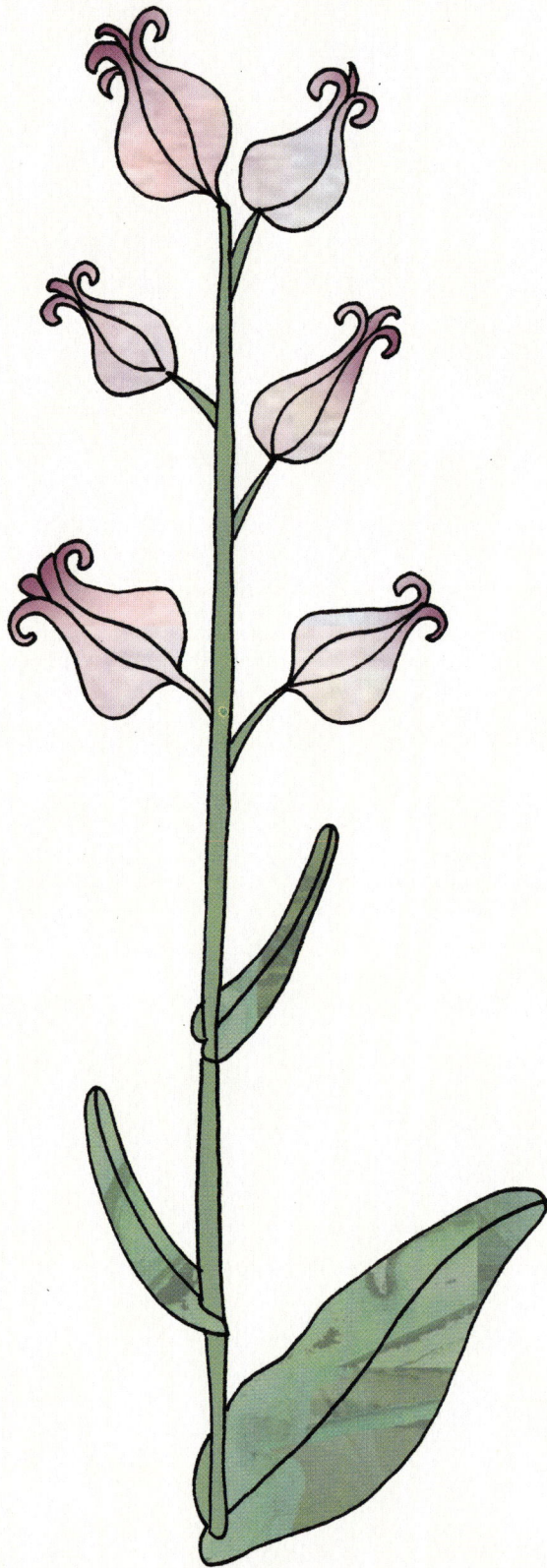

Lyreleaf Jewelflower

Streptanthus carinatus

Appearance: This slender wildflower is similar to Gordon's bladderpod in that it is a sign of the upcoming spring. This plant grows lobed, lance-shaped, green leaves and the stems are thin and long, growing up to 30 inches (76 cm) tall. It has unique, small, vase-shaped flowers about ½ inch (1 cm) long with each of the four petals coming together and curling on the ends. The flowers range from white to yellow to maroon. Its fruits are green, flat seed pods that can be up to 3 inches (7.5 cm) long and point upward along the stem.

Habitat: Only found in southern Arizona, southern New Mexico, and west Texas between 2,000 and 5,500 feet (610 and 1,676 m) elevation in canyons, washes, and rocky slopes.

Blooming season: February through April.

Lifespan: Annual.

Environmental role: The flowers are a nectar source for native pollinators and the seeds are eaten by birds and small mammals. These plants also help prevent soil erosion.

Foraging: No known foraging uses.

Plant friends: Arizona jewelflower.

Palmer's Agave

Agave palmeri

Appearance: Agaves are a typical desert plant, resilient and spiky with a nostalgic look. This succulent is a basal rosette (a circular arrangement of leaves growing close to the ground from the base of a plant's stem) of stiff, swordlike, spine-tipped leaves with a distinct pale bluish-green color. This rosette can grow up to 4 feet (1.2 m) tall. It grows a very tall, thick flower stalk with yellow leaves on the end that can grow up to 20 feet (6 m).

Habitat: Frost-hardy and slow growing, it's found in Arizona and New Mexico between 3,500 and 7,500 feet (1,067 and 2,286 m) elevation on rocky, open slopes with lots of sunlight. Chaparral and grassland biomes.

Blooming season: May through August.

Lifespan: Five to twenty-five years. Nicknamed the "century plant" because people used to think it flowered once every one hundred years, but this plant only blooms once near the end of its life, after which the entire plant dies.

Environmental role: This agave plays a vital role in the ecology of its habitat. It stands as a symbol of resilience in the harsh desert as it can adapt to extreme climate conditions. Its looming flowers give nectar to hummingbirds and bats. It has long been of great benefit to humans (see Foraging). It is a tenacious plant that helps prevent erosion with its complicated root system. Scientists have been studying this plant as a source for bioenergy.

Foraging: Indigenous peoples have used "century plants" widely for food, beverages, fiber, soap, and medicine for thousands of years and still do today. I personally have not foraged agave, but benefit from consuming agave syrup, pulque, mescal, and more. The process of making food and beverages from agave is very involved with many different steps.

Plant friends: Any Agavaceae like the Arizona agave are relatives of this plant and are often seen growing near soaptree yucca.

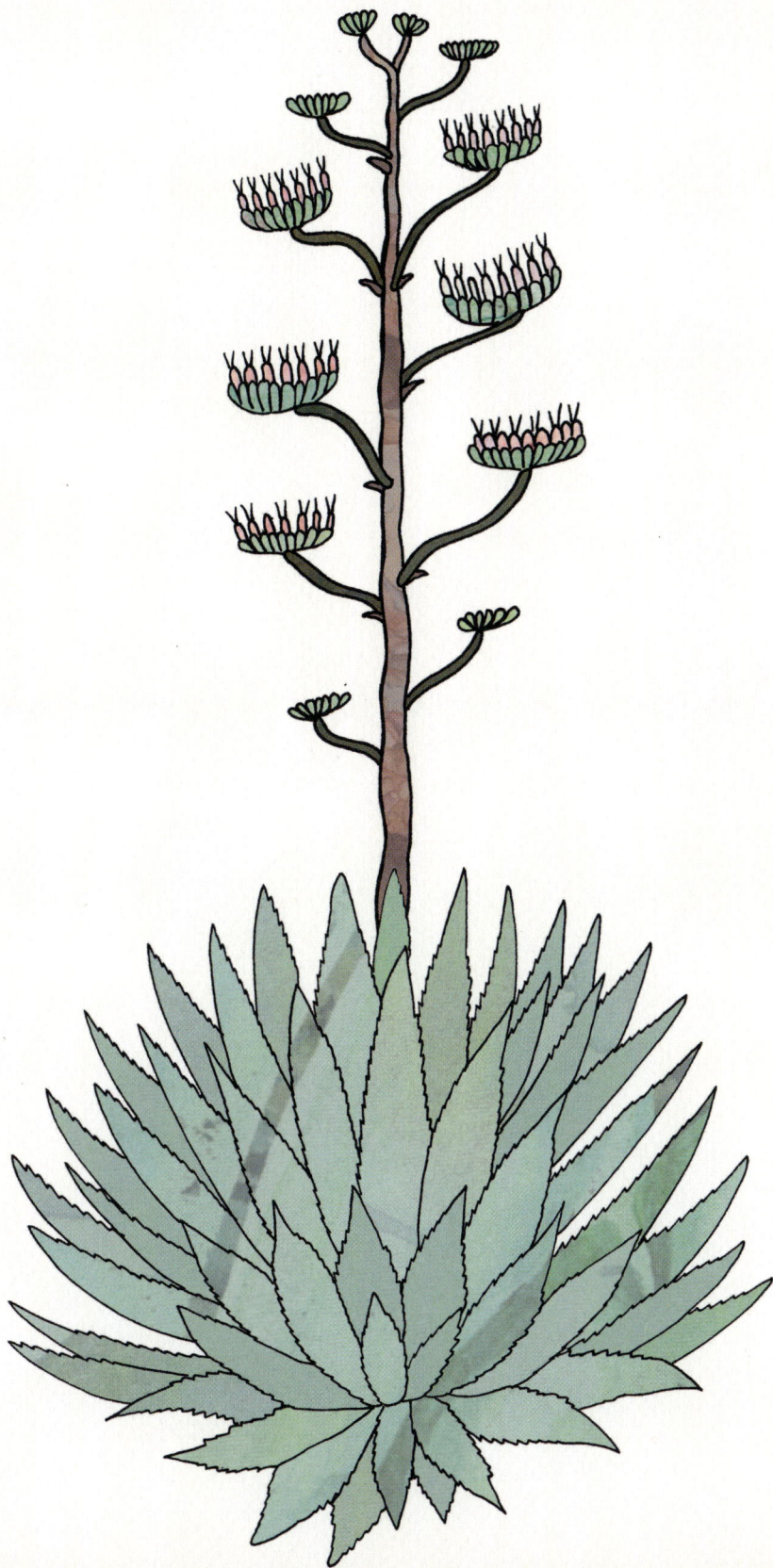

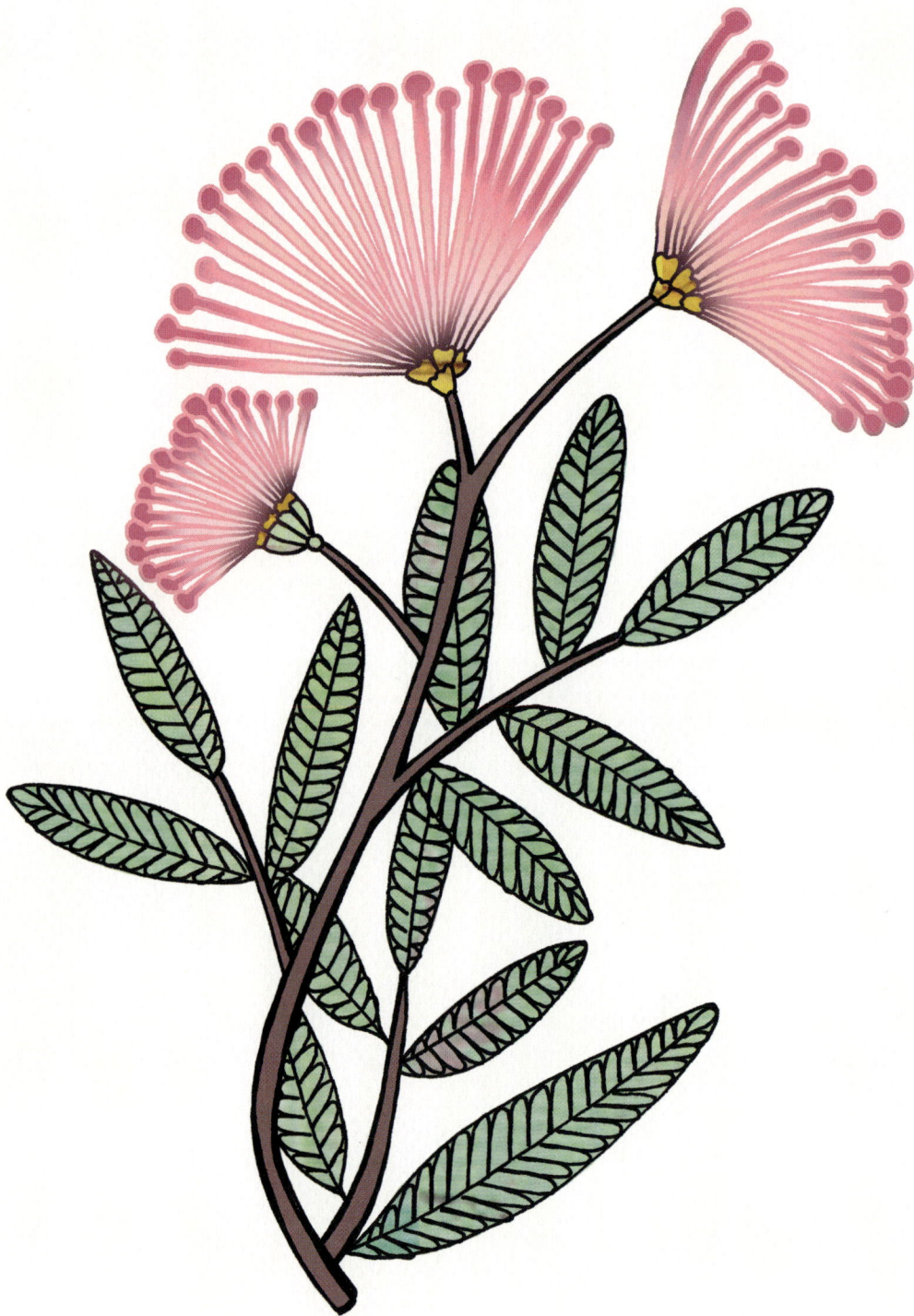

Pink Fairy Duster

Calliandra eriophylla

Appearance: This magical, short desert shrub is straggly and densely branched, growing up to 3 feet (91 cm) tall and 3 feet (91 cm) wide. It has small fernlike leaves but is most well known for its beautiful, fluffy, ball-shaped pink flowers that are made of twenty or more thin filaments emerging from small, clustered flowers. These bushes look like they are covered in a pink mist when in full bloom.

Habitat: Southwestern United States and Northern Mexico below 5,000 feet (1,524 m) on hillsides, desert washes, and slopes.

Blooming season: February through July.

Lifespan: Can live up to ten years.

Environmental role: Pink fairy duster's scruffy shape offers shelter and nesting sites to small desert wildlife. Its attractive flowers offer a vital nectar source for pollinators like hummingbirds and butterflies and its seeds are an important food for small mammals and birds like quail. It also has a dense root structure that helps stabilize the soil. It is a symbol of endurance in the desert because it blooms even in arid conditions. Many Southwestern Indigenous peoples have used fairy duster medicinally for thousands of years.

Foraging: This mystical pink flower is often used in flower essences (aqueous extracts) as it can calm the nervous system and promote tranquility. It is also known to have anti-inflammatory properties and native Yavapai people used it as a gynecological aid after childbirth. I like to decorate cakes and salads with these flowers to add some fairy magic.

Plant friends: Baja fairy duster.

Santa Catalina Prairie Clover

Dalea pulchra

Appearance: This rare gem is an upright, short, woody shrub that can grow up to 3 feet (91 cm) tall with brown stems. Each stem hosts about five to seven tiny, grayish-green leaves that are covered in silky hairs. It has small, pealike, purple and white flower petals that surround a spherical, fuzzy white spike. Santa Catalina prairie clovers also have a soft, fragrant scent.

Habitat: Only found in southern Arizona and southern New Mexico between 2,000 and 5,000 feet (610 and 1,524 m) elevation in grasslands, rocky slopes, and canyons. Most abundant in the Santa Catalina and Rincon mountains near Tucson, Arizona.

Blooming season: February through July.

Lifespan: Several years, though its exact lifespan is unknown.

Environmental role: This shrub is important to the desert grasslands because it offers nitrogen fixation: nitrogen-fixing bacteria in the roots of the plant that help convert atmospheric nitrogen into ammonia which is readily absorbed by organisms in the soil. Its flowers feed many native pollinators, its seeds feed small animals, and it is a host for butterfly larvae. Its tough structure and drought-tolerant nature lets it withstand storms, wind, and other disturbances, making it a great native option for landscaping in the desert.

Foraging: This specific type of prairie clover does not have any known uses, but prairie clover leaves have been used to make tea to pour on wounds and to treat illnesses like diarrhea and pneumonia. Prairie clover teas can also be taken to strengthen the heart before exercise.

Plant friends: Purple prairie clover, Parry's false prairie clover, white prairie clover, and soft prairie clover.

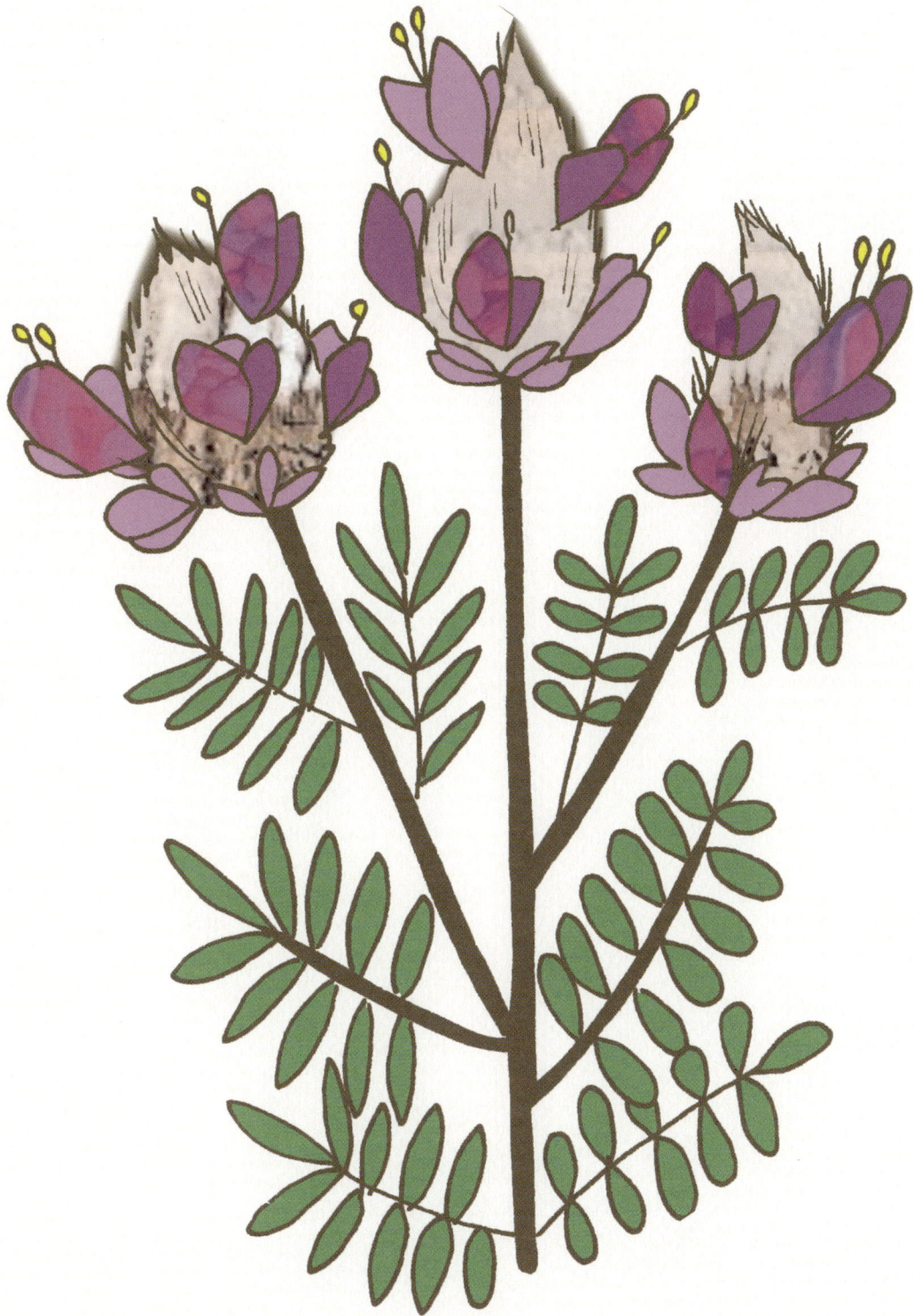

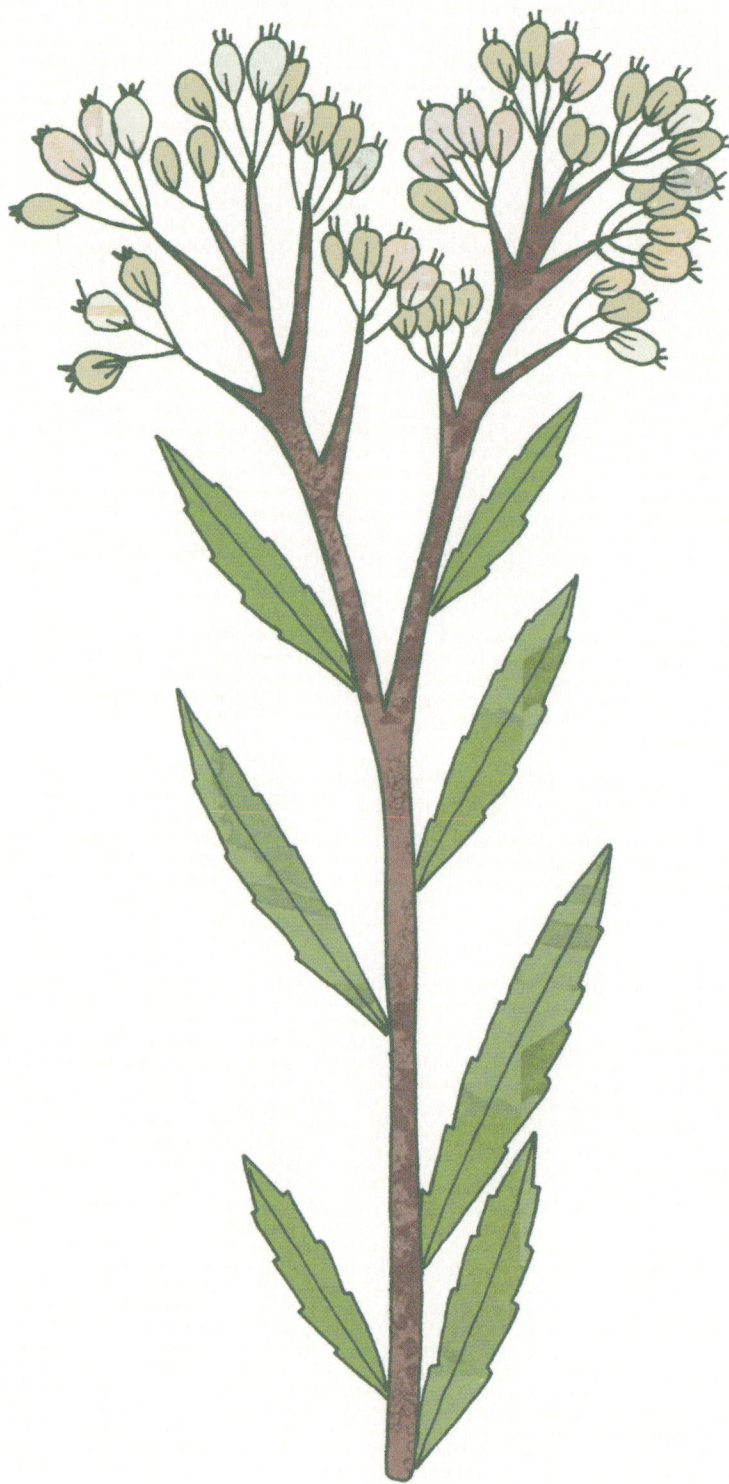

Seepwillow

Baccharis salicifolia

Appearance: This pollinator favorite is mostly found in riparian areas throughout the Sonoran Desert. Seepwillow is a tall shrub that forms thickets and grows up to 10 feet (3 m) tall. The stems secrete a yellowish resin that makes the fine hairs on them sticky. The new stems—green, at first, before turning brown—spread horizontally before becoming erect and are covered with lance-shaped, willowlike, green leaves that can be up to 6 inches (15 cm) long. Seepwillow is most recognizable for its small, cream-colored, fuzzy flowers that grow in clusters at the ends of its stems. Once the flowers have dried, they release seeds that are topped with the fluff from the flower and are spread by the wind.

Habitat: Found in the Southwestern United States, all of Mexico, and parts of South America at elevations up to 5,500 feet (1,676 m) in moist wetlands, near springs, riparian woodlands, dry washes, and disturbed areas.

Blooming season: February through October.

Lifespan: Can live up to twenty years in ideal conditions.

Environmental role: Seepwillow blooms almost throughout the entire year, making it essential for pollinators, like native bees, which will often be found covering the plants. It is also a host plant for butterfly larvae, and its seeds are consumed by birds and small mammals. A large range of Indigenous peoples have used seepwillow medicinally throughout time.

Foraging: An infusion of the leaves can be used to encourage hair growth and to treat wounds and insect bites (as used by many Indigenous peoples). Seepwillow has antibacterial properties, as I have found most resinous desert plants do. I have not personally used this plant yet but hope to at some point.

Plant friends: Desert broom and Roosevelt weed.

Teddy Bear Cholla

Cylindropuntia bigelovii

Appearance: Teddy bear cholla, also known as jumping cholla, is a well-known desert cactus. It is a slow-growing, treelike cactus that can grow up to 6 feet (1.8 m) tall. It has a trunk and many thick, stubby green branches that are completely covered in formidable, sharp, slightly hooked, cream-colored spines—giving it a fuzzy, teddy-bear look. As the arms are easily detachable and their spines cling to anything that brushes up against them, there will often be arms spread out all around the ground near the main cactus's vicinity. From personal experience, these cacti can really hurt when they come in contact with skin and are very hard to remove without becoming further entangled in spines. These cacti produce waxy, pale-yellow or pale-green flowers about 1.5 inches (3.8 cm) across that close up at night.

Habitat: Found in the Mojave and Sonoran Deserts up to 3,000 feet (914 m) elevation in sandy flats, rocky washes, hillsides, and desert mountains.

Blooming season: March through June.

Lifespan: Can live up to twenty years.

Environmental role: Their dense, thick, spined branches provide protection from predators for birds and small mammals, and they support a variety of other desert plants nearby. The cholla flowers produce nectar that feeds pollinators like solitary native bees, who also take shelter inside the flowers at night—the sight of the flowers closed around the sleeping bees is adorable. This cactus (like most cacti) stores water in its branches so it can survive through periods of drought and its limbs propagate easily, making it very resilient and widespread. The Tohono O'odham have eaten cholla flower buds for thousands of years, enjoying an excellent source of electrolytes and vitamins.

Foraging: The flower buds (before the flowers open) can be very carefully collected to be cooked and eaten. First, use creosote stems to brush the spines off the buds, then carefully remove the buds with sticks or tongs. The fresh buds can be boiled and either eaten right away or dried and rehydrated later. They are full of electrolytes, and I believe eating cacti regularly can extend our lives.

Plant friends: Staghorn cholla and Christmas cholla.

Cholla Removal Tools

Cholla, and especially teddy bear cholla, can be particularly hard to remove from skin and clothing, which is why it is important to watch where you are walking so you don't accidentally brush up against or walk through any. It's also smart to wear pants and closed-toe shoes when hiking in the desert. Here are some simple tools you can use to remove a piece of cholla if it's unfortunately attached itself to you:

- Tweezers—I carry a pair on me at all times.

- A large comb is probably the best tool for this as it can remove them with one swipe.

- No tools with you? Two sticks will do the job!

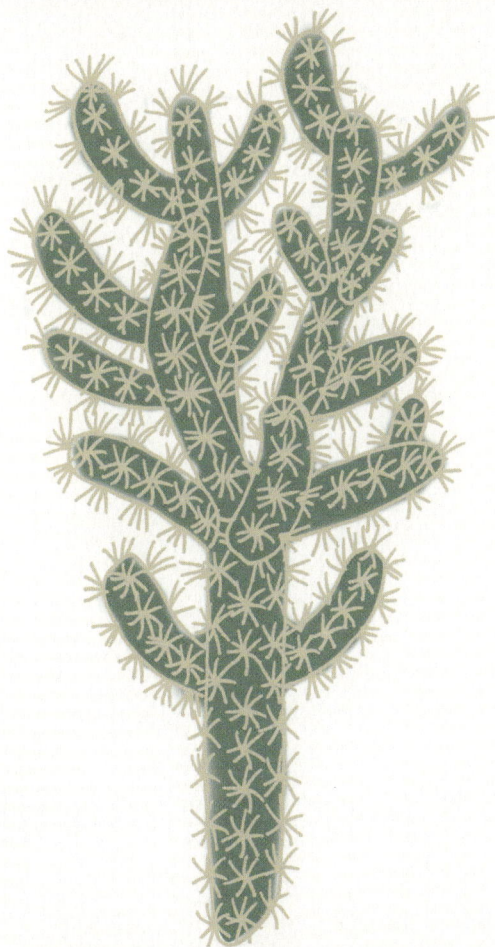

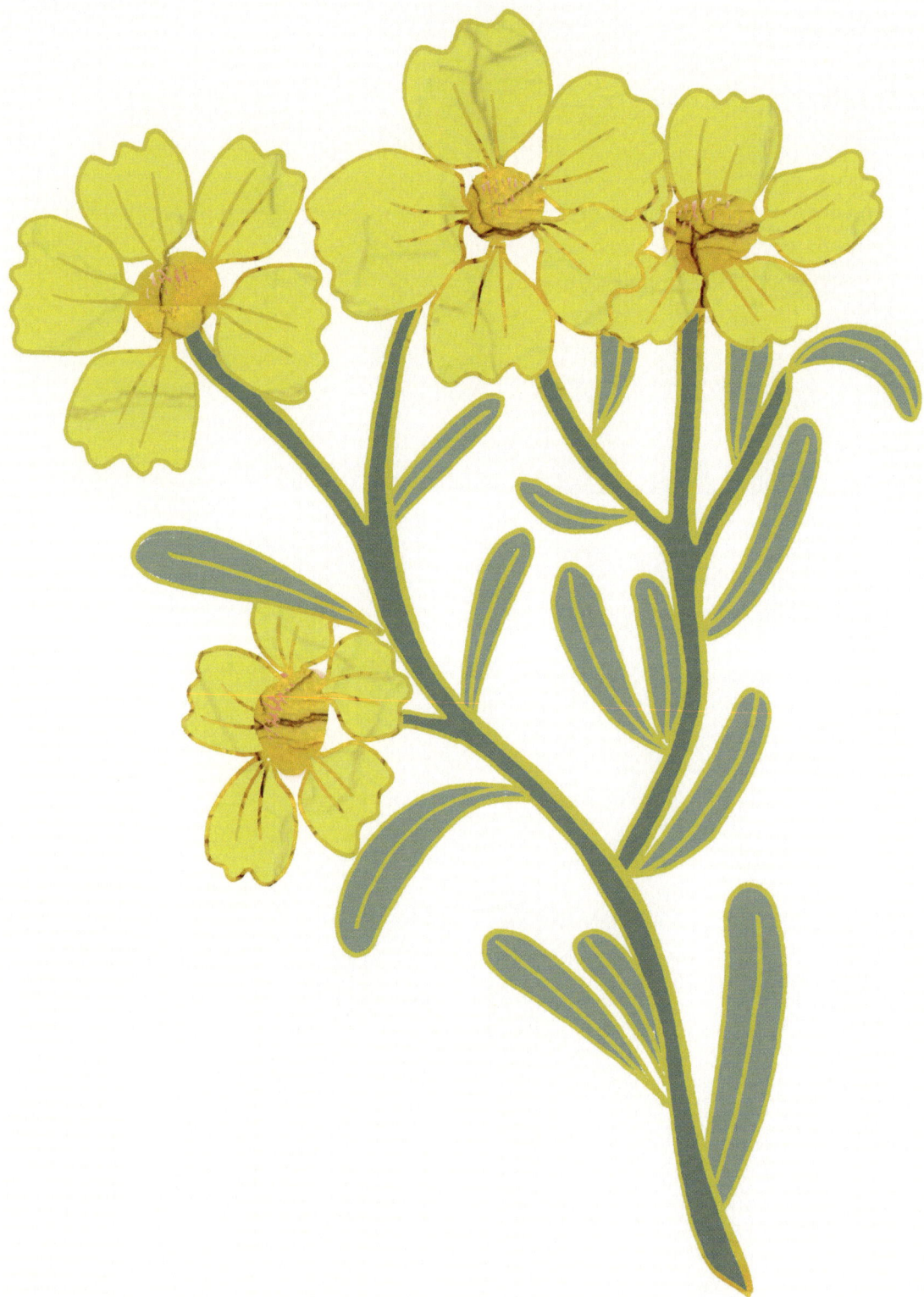

Whitestem Paperflower

Psilostrophe cooperi

Appearance: This small, rounded herb can grow up to 2 feet (61 cm) tall with white, woolly stems and narrow, linear green leaves. One showy yellow flower, about 1 inch (2.5 cm) across, sits at the end of each stem. The three to six flower rays look dry and papery and stay on the plant long after they have lost their yellow color, giving the plant its common name.

Habitat: Found in the Sonoran and Mojave Deserts between 2,000 and 6,000 feet (610 and 1,829 m) elevation in lower and upper deserts, rocky hillsides, mesas, plains, and sandy washes.

Blooming season: February through September.

Lifespan: Perennial, living for more than two years.

Environmental role: Whitestem paperflower plays a crucial role in the desert ecosystem by providing nectar for pollinators and seeds for birds and small mammals throughout a large portion of the year. It also provides ground cover for small insects, reptiles, and mammals. This plant also has a lot of medicinal uses.

Foraging: Whitestem paperflower would be a great addition to any tea or salve as it has antibacterial, anti-inflammatory, antifungal, and antiviral properties! It is a powerful plant and should be incorporated more often into natural medicines.

Plant friends: Desert zinnia and desert marigold (any plants in the Asteraceae family).

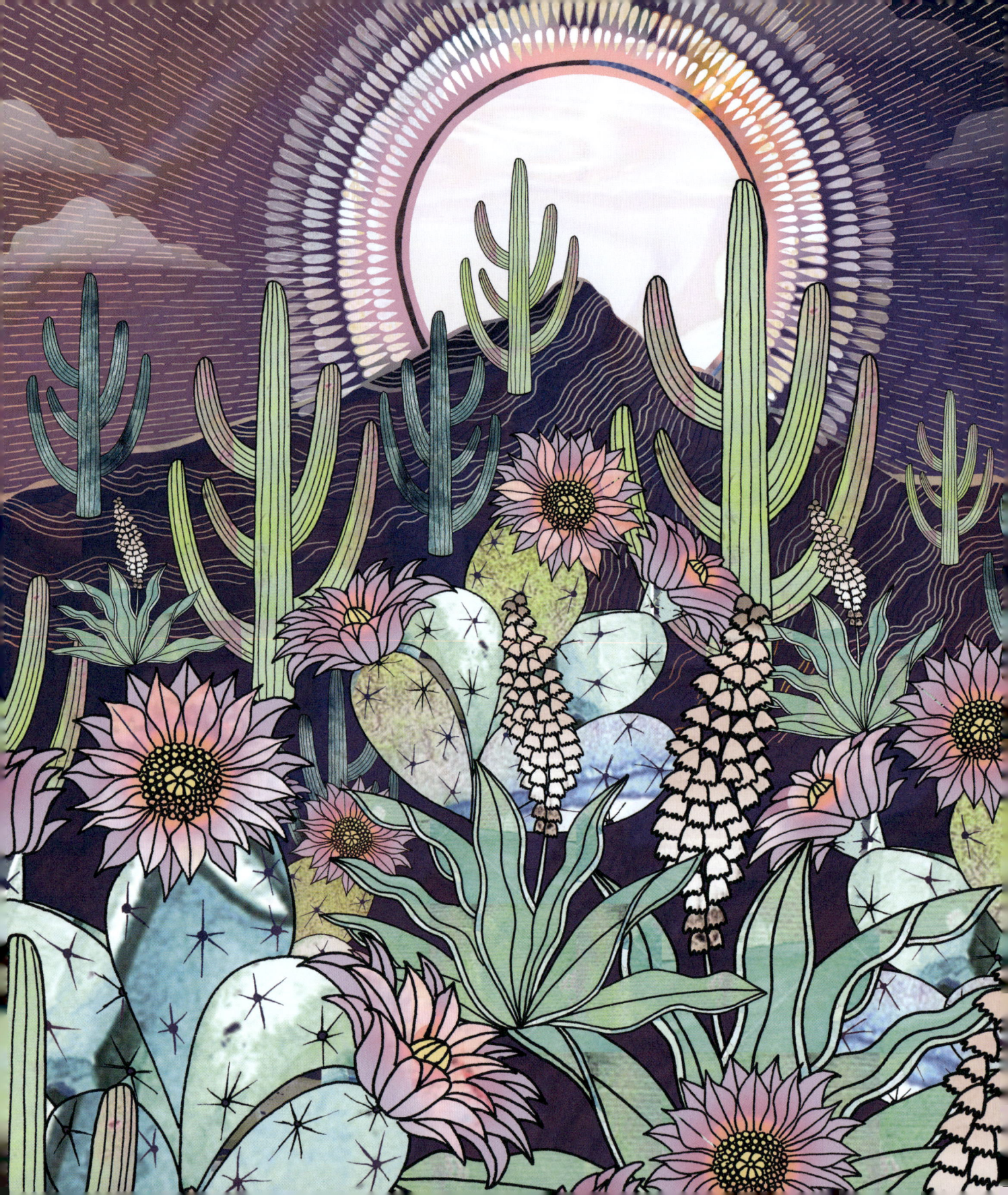

Conclusion

After writing this book and reflecting, I find my heart swelling with an even deeper gratitude, not only for the Sonoran Desert but for nature in all its forms. If we look closely enough, we can see the delicate interconnections between ourselves, the land, and the plants that call this place home. The fiery sunsets, the bold cacti, the deep valleys, and the towering mountains all beckon us, yearning for a reciprocal bond. Yet, I am often disheartened by the relentless march of urbanization, which has scarred so much of our wild lands, erasing ecosystems without regard for plants and wildlife—the very lifelines we must learn to honor and depend upon. When profit becomes the priority, everything else falters.

But glimmers of hope shine through, like rays of light piercing the dark. In the faces of those who work to preserve and restore this desert—like the Sky Island Alliance and the Tucson Wildlife Center—I see a shared vision. These individuals, defying the narrow teachings of a society obsessed with consumption, choose understanding, compassion, and connection.

As the years pass and I spend more time in the Arizona desert, I have come to realize that when I give to the earth, it returns in abundance. I feel the land's sorrow during droughts, grieve for the desert lost to development, and mourn the wildflowers poisoned by chemicals. Yet, I am forever embraced and protected by these desert plant beings. My heart aches for the land, but I also know that the universe moves through love. I can only focus on the light I can offer, in the hope it might ignite others.

With this book, my aim is simple: to spark curiosity and aid in fostering a continuous relationship with the desert and its abundance. I believe that connecting with nature through any of our senses enriches our lives, deepening our empathy for the natural world and helping us understand ourselves. If we build sustainable relationships with plants, we can learn to live in harmony rather than domination. Slowly, we can unlearn the individualism and greed that have defined our lives, paving the way for a future where values outshine personal gain.

Thank you for reading and for experiencing the Sonoran Desert through my Rosie lens.

Glossary

Annual: A plant that blooms once every year, with a lifecycle of a year.

Biennial: A plant that blooms every two years.

Biodiversity: The variety of life in a particular habitat or ecosystem, including species diversity, genetic diversity, and ecosystem diversity.

Biome: A large ecological area characterized by specific climate conditions and the organisms adapted to those conditions (e.g., forests, deserts, grasslands).

Bosques: The Spanish word for "forests"; often refers to specific ecosystems or forest types in certain regions, like the "mesquite bosques" in the Southwestern US.

Caliche: A hard, white, chalky layer of soil or rock formed by the accumulation of calcium carbonate.

Camphor: A white, aromatic substance derived from the wood of the camphor tree.

Cochineal: A small, parasitic insect whose dried bodies are used to produce carmine dye, which is often used in cosmetics, textile dye, and food.

Distiller: A device that purifies liquids, especially alcohol, through distillation (heating and cooling).

Flora: The collective term for all plant life in a particular region or environment.

Germinate: To begin to grow or develop, typically referring to seeds sprouting into plants.

Hemiparasitic: A type of parasitic plant that partially depends on a host for nutrients but still carries out photosynthesis.

Herbaceous: Describing plants that have soft, nonwoody stems, typically dying back at the end of the growing season.

Herbal: Relating to herbs or plants, especially those used for medicinal purposes.

Hydrosol: A water-based solution obtained by distilling plants, often used in herbalism or aromatherapy.

Invasive: Referring to non-native species that cause harm to the environment, economy, or human health by spreading rapidly.

Keystone species: A species that has a disproportionately large effect on its ecosystem relative to its abundance or biomass, often playing a critical role in maintaining ecological balance.

Legume: A plant in the pea family, which typically has pods containing seeds; known for its ability to fix nitrogen in the soil.

Mesa: A flat-topped mountain or hill with steep sides, typically found in arid regions.

Monsoon: A seasonal wind pattern that brings heavy rains, often in tropical and subtropical regions (like the Sonoran Desert).

Mordanted: Treated with a mordant (a substance that fixes dye) to ensure that a dye adheres to a fabric or other material.

Nitrogen fixation: The process by which certain plants, like legumes, convert nitrogen gas from the atmosphere into a form that can be used by plants for growth.

Oxymel: A traditional medicinal syrup made from honey, vinegar, and herbs often used for its soothing properties.

Palmately: Describing a leaf shape where the leaflets or veins spread out from a common point, resembling fingers on a hand.

Perennial: A plant that lives for more than two years, often flowering and producing seeds multiple times in its lifespan.

Petrichor: The pleasant, earthy scent produced when rain falls on dry soil or ground, caused by the release of certain oils and compounds.

Pollinators: Organisms (like bees, butterflies, and birds) that transfer pollen from one flower to another, facilitating plant reproduction; critical for many food crops.

Poultice: A soft, moist mass of material (often made from herbs or clay) applied to the skin to relieve pain or inflammation.

Propagate: To reproduce or spread plants, animals, or organisms, often through methods like cuttings or seeds.

Rosette: A circular arrangement of leaves or petals, typically at the base of a plant.

Prostrate: Lying flat or growing along the ground; often used to describe plants that spread out rather than grow upright.

Riparian zone: The area of land adjacent to a river, stream, or other waterbody. It plays a crucial role in maintaining the health of the ecosystem, as it helps to filter water, prevent erosion, and provide habitat for various plants and animals. Riparian zones typically have vegetation that is adapted to moist conditions, and they act as a buffer between the land and the water, supporting biodiversity and promoting water quality.

Semiparasitic: A type of parasitic plant that relies on a host for water and nutrients but which can also photosynthesize.

Sky islands: Isolated mountain ranges that rise above surrounding desert areas, often hosting unique ecosystems.

Soil erosion: The process by which soil is worn away by wind, water, or human activity, leading to a loss of fertile soil.

Spines: Sharp, pointed structures found on some plants, like cacti, used for defense or water conservation.

Weeds: Unwanted plants that grow aggressively and can harm cultivated crops, ecosystems, or landscapes (native plants are not weeds).

Tincture: A concentrated herbal extract made by soaking plants in alcohol or another solvent.

Xeriscaping: Landscaping designed to reduce the need for water, often by using drought-tolerant plants and efficient water management practices.

Sources

Abad, Maria José, and Paulina Bermejo. "Baccharis (Compositae): A Review Update." Accessed October 5, 2024. www.arkat-usa.org/get-file/19602/

American Southwest. "Plant Index." Accessed August 2024. https://www.americansouthwest.net/plants/index.html

"Arizona Agave (Agave × arizonica)." Save Plants. Last modified August 8, 2024. https://saveplants.org/plant-profile/44/Agave-x-arizonica/Arizona-Agave/

Arizona Department of Education. "Saguaro Fun Facts." Accessed August 15, 2024. https://www.azed.gov/sites/default/files/2019/02/Saguaro%20Fun%20Facts.pdf

Arizona Native Plant Society. "New Mexico Thistle." August 28, 2021. https://aznps.com/2021/02/28/new-mexico-thistle/

Arizona-Sonora Desert Museum. "Sonoran Desert Fact Sheets." Accessed August 2024. https://www.desertmuseum.org/kids/oz/long-fact-sheets/

Arizonensis. "California Mistletoe (Phoradendron californicum)." Arizonensis. Accessed August 2, 2024. http://www.arizonensis.org/sonoran/fieldguide/plantae/phoradendron_calif.html

"Arrow Weed Plant." Ethnoherbalist. Accessed August 11, 2024. https://www.ethnoherbalist.com/southern-california-native-plants-medicinal/arrow-weed-plant/

"The Benefits of California Poppy." The Herbal Academy. Last modified December 10, 2021. https://theherbalacademy.com/blog/california-poppy-benefits/?srsltid=AfmBOoqXXzcr7vbjyvXQ_THD44zt0b4pTnWWlgWExHsh8i5ATUTHkYet

Botanical Realm. "Desert Purple Mat (Nama demissa)." Accessed August 23, 2024. https://www.botanicalrealm.com/plant-identification/desert-purple-mat-nama-demissa-demissa/

"California Poppy." Encyclopaedia Britannica. Last modified January 11, 2023. https://www.britannica.com/plant/California-poppy

Calscape. "Find Native Plants." Accessed August 2024. https://calscape.org

Center for Plant Conservation. "Peniocereus greggii var. transmontanus (Desert Night-Blooming Cereus)." Accessed August 24, 2024. https://saveplants.org/plant-profile/14387/Peniocereus-greggii-var.-transmontanus/Desert-Night-blooming-Cereus/

"Desert Ironwood Tree." Ironwood Forest National Monument. Accessed August 21, 2024. https://ironwoodforest.org/about/the-monument/learn/desert-ironwood-tree/

"Desert Lavender." Arizona Municipal Water Users Association (AMWUA). Accessed August 11, 2024. https://www.amwua.org/plants/desert-lavender

Dunbar Spring Neighborhood Foresters. "Plant Resources." Last modified August 2, 2024. https://dunbarspringneighborhoodforesters.org/plant-resources/

Earth Notions. "Wolfberry Jam Recipe." Earth Notions. Accessed August 2, 2024. https://www.earthnotions.com/recipe/wolfberry-jam

Firefly Forest. "Southeastern Arizona Wildflowers and Plants." Accessed August 2, 2024. https://www.fireflyforest.com/flowers/

Gardenia. "Plant Finder." Accessed August 2, 2024. https://www.gardenia.net/plant-finder#

"Globemallow: Binding the Desert's Wounds." PBS SoCal. Accessed August 11, 2024. https://www.pbssocal.org/redefine/globemallow-binding-the-deserts-wounds

Hernandez, Javier. "Desert Broom: Another Medicinal Plant." *Arizona Daily Independent,* April 26, 2015. https://arizonadailyindependent.com/2015/04/26/desert-broom-another-medicinal-plant/amp/

Lady Bird Johnson Wildflower Center. "Find Plants." Accessed August 2024. https://www.wildflower.org/plants/

Legacy Wilderness Academy. "Desert Hackberry." Legacy Wilderness Academy. Accessed August 2, 2024. https://www.legacywildernessacademy.com/blog/desert-hackberry

Mexican Food Journal. "Cactus Fruit Pico de Gallo." Mexican Food Journal. Accessed August 2, 2024. https://mexicanfoodjournal.com/cactus-fruit-pico-de-gallo/

My Herbal Box. "Ocotillo Medicine: The Mover and Shaker." My Herbal Box. Last modified March 9, 2023. https://www.myherbalbox.com/blogs/in-the-weeds/ocotillo-medicine-the-mover-and-shaker

National Park Service. "Sonoran Desert Ecosystems." National Park Service. Last modified January 25, 2022. Accessed August 7, 2024. https://www.nps.gov/im/sodn/ecosystems.htm

Native Seeds/Search. "Hopi Red Dye Amaranth." Native Seeds/Search. Accessed August 8, 2024. https://www.nativeseeds.org/pages/hopi-red-dye-amaranth

Nature Collective. "Plant Guide." Accessed August 2, 2024. https://naturecollective.org/plant-guide/

The Nature Conservancy. "Wings & Water: Wetland Producers." The Nature Conservancy, January 2019. https://www.nature.org/content/dam/tnc/nature/en/documents/UT_WingsWater_WetlandProducers_Jan19.pdf

Permaculture. "Thistles: A Highly Nutritious and Medicinal Weed." Permaculture, September 18, 2020. https://www.permaculture.co.uk/articles/thistles-a-highly-nutritious-and-medicinal-weed/

Pitchstone Waters. "Creosote Bush: An Unassuming but Ancient Form of Life All Around Us." Accessed August 23, 2024. https://www.pitchstonewaters.com/creosote-bush-an-unassuming-but-ancient-form-of-life-all-around-us/

Prickly Petals. "Agave palmeri: Revealing the Distinct Ecological Importance and Sustainability Potential." Last modified August 11, 2024. https://pricklypetals.com/agave-palmeri-revealing-the-distinct-ecological-importance-and-sustainability-potential/?feed_id=15296&_unique_id=654ae8861ed8c&utm_source=Medium&utm_medium=admin&utm_campaign=FS+Poster

Southwest Desert Flora. "Index." Accessed August 2024. https://southwestdesertflora.com/index.html

Theodore Payne Foundation. "Abutilon palmeri (Palmer's Abutilon)." Theodore Payne Foundation. Accessed August 2, 2024. https://theodorepayne.org/nativeplantdatabase/index.php?title=Abutilon_palmeri

Tohono O'odham Nation. "Tohono O'odham History." Tohono O'odham Nation. Accessed August 11, 2024. http://www.tonation-nsn.gov/tohono-oodham-history/

U.S. Fish and Wildlife Service. "California Least Tern (Sterna antillarum browni)." Environmental Conservation Online System (ECOS). Accessed August 7, 2024. https://ecos.fws.gov/ecp/species/1702

U.S. Forest Service. "Datura Wrightii (Sacred Datura)." U.S. Forest Service. Accessed August 2, 2024. https://www.fs.usda.gov/wildflowers/beauty/Sky_Islands/plants/Datura_wrightii/index.shtml

University of Arizona. "Campus Arboretum." Accessed August 11, 2024. https://apps.cals.arizona.edu/arboretum/taxon.aspx?id=67

Western Native Seed. "Fesca Ripa Plant Guide." Last modified August 25, 2024. https://www.westernnativeseed.com/plant%20guides/fesaripg.pdf

Index

Recipes by Season

Autumn

Spring

Summer

Winter

Blooms by Month

January

February

March

April

Gordon's Bladderpod, 160
Graham's Nipple Cactus, 74
Littleleaf Rhatany, 37
Lyreleaf Jewelflower, 163
Mexican Manzanita, 122
New Mexico Thistle, 69
Ocotillo, 41
Palmer's Indian Mallow, 125
Parry's Penstemon, 45
Pink Fairy Duster, 167
Purple Mat, 49
Purple Three-awn Grass, 126
Sacred Datura, 87
Saguaro, 50
Santa Catalina Prairie Clover, 168
Santa Rita Prickly Pear Cactus, 46
Seepwillow, 171
Soaptree Yucca, 91
Southern Cattail, 134
Southwestern Prickly Poppy, 92
Staghorn Cholla, 53
Tansyleaf Tansyaster, 139
Teddy Bear Cholla, 172
Velvet Mesquite Tree, 77
Whitestem Paperflower, 175
Yellow Palo Verde, 42

May

Angelita Daisy, 97
Arizona Agave, 143
Arizona Hedgehog Cactus, 19
Arizona Lupine, 20
Arizona Thistle, 101
Arrowweed, 144
Big Saltbush, 107
Blackfoot Daisy, 23
Brittlebush, 24
California Buckwheat, 108
Catclaw Acacia, 112
Chuparosa, 148
Cleftleaf Wild Heliotrope, 29
Cowpen Daisy, 63
Desert Evening Primrose, 151
Desert Globemallow, 32
Desert Hackberry, 115
Desert Ironwood Tree, 34
Desert Lavender, 30
Desert Milkweed, 116
Desert Senna, 66
Desert Thistle, 69
Desert Willow, 70
Engelmann Prickly Pear Cactus, 82
Firewheel, 73
Fiveneedle Pricklyleaf, 155
Fremont Wolfberry, 156
Gordon's Bladderpod, 160

Graham's Nipple Cactus, 74
Littleleaf Rhatany, 37
Mexican Manzanita, 122
New Mexico Thistle, 69
Ocotillo, 41
Palmer's Agave, 164
Palmer's Indian Mallow, 125
Parry's Penstemon, 45
Pink Fairy Duster, 167
Purple Mat, 49
Purple Three-awn Grass, 126
Sacred Datura, 87
Saguaro, 50
Santa Catalina Prairie Clover, 168
Santa Rita Prickly Pear Cactus, 46
Seepwillow, 171
Silverleaf Nightshade, 133
Soaptree Yucca, 91
Southern Cattail, 134
Southwestern Prickly Poppy, 92
Staghorn Cholla, 53
Tansyleaf Tansyaster, 139
Teddy Bear Cholla, 172
Velvet Mesquite Tree, 77
Whitestem Paperflower, 175
Yellow Palo Verde, 42

June

Angelita Daisy, 97
Arizona Agave, 143
Arizona Poppy, 60
Arizona Thistle, 101
Arrowweed, 144
Big Saltbush, 107
Blackfoot Daisy, 23
California Buckwheat, 108
Catclaw Acacia, 112
Chuparosa, 148
Cleftleaf Wild Heliotrope, 29
Cowpen Daisy, 63
Desert Evening Primrose, 151
Desert Globemallow, 32
Desert Horsepurslane, 84
Desert Ironwood Tree, 34
Desert Lavender, 30
Desert Milkweed, 116
Desert Senna, 66
Desert Thistle, 69
Desert Willow, 70
Engelmann Prickly Pear Cactus, 82
February, 49
Firewheel, 73
Fishhook Barrel Cactus, 118
Fiveneedle Pricklyleaf, 155
Graham's Nipple Cactus, 74
Littleleaf Rhatany, 37

Mt. Lemmon Marigold, 78
New Mexico Thistle, 69
Night-Blooming Cereus, 81
Ocotillo, 41
Palmer's Agave, 164
Palmer's Indian Mallow, 125
Pink Fairy Duster, 167
Purple Three-awn Grass, 126
Sacred Datura, 87
Saguaro, 50
Saguaro Fruit, 88
Santa Catalina Prairie Clover, 168
Santa Rita Prickly Pear Cactus, 46
Seepwillow, 171
Silverleaf Nightshade, 133
Soaptree Yucca, 91
Southern Cattail, 134
Southwestern Prickly Poppy, 92
Staghorn Cholla, 53
Tansyleaf Tansyaster, 139
Teddy Bear Cholla, 172
Velvet Mesquite Tree, 77
Whitestem Paperflower, 175
Wild Sunflower, 136

July

Angelita Daisy, 97
Arizona Agave, 143
Arizona Poppy, 60
Arizona Thistle, 101
Arrowweed, 144
Big Saltbush, 107
Blackfoot Daisy, 23
California Buckwheat, 108
Cardinal Flower, 111
Catclaw Acacia, 112
Chuparosa, 148
Cowpen Daisy, 63
Desert Globemallow, 32
Desert Horsepurslane, 84
Desert Lavender, 30
Desert Milkweed, 116
Desert Senna, 66
Desert Thistle, 69
Desert Willow, 70
Engelmann Prickly Pear Cactus, 82
February, 49
Firewheel, 73
Fishhook Barrel Cactus, 118
Fiveneedle Pricklyleaf, 155
Graham's Nipple Cactus, 74
Hopi Red Dye Amaranth, 59
Littleleaf Rhatany, 37
Mexican Manzanita, 122
Mt. Lemmon Marigold, 78
New Mexico Thistle, 69

Acknowledgments

To my mother, Kathleen, who was a writer, a feminist, a lover of the moon. She lost the battle to her depression and committed suicide many years ago. She would be so proud to learn where I am in accomplishing my goals, creating a happy existence and writing this book.

To my father, Chris, who I recently met and have built a great relationship with based off our shared love of the desert.

To my sister Ariel, who was a published writer, a singer, and a photographer. She passed away too young, but I know she would be celebrating my wins and pushing me forward.

To my brother Aaron, who was my best friend growing up. He also passed away too young. We experienced much hardship and happiness together. I am grateful to have known him and his sensitive nature.

To my best friends, Gabi and Lauren, who continually support me in so many ways and whom I can share my passions with.

To my employees, who really are the best out there. I wouldn't be able to do all I do without them.

To my creative community here in Tucson, Arizona, who have shown me the importance of finding and fostering relationships with like-minded people. Without community I am but a fraction of myself.

And of course, to the enchanting Sonoran Desert and all the magical plants that I have built relationships with over the years. I have learned so much from them and am offered peace through them on a daily basis. I have never felt so grounded and connected and I owe it all to the Sonoran Desert.

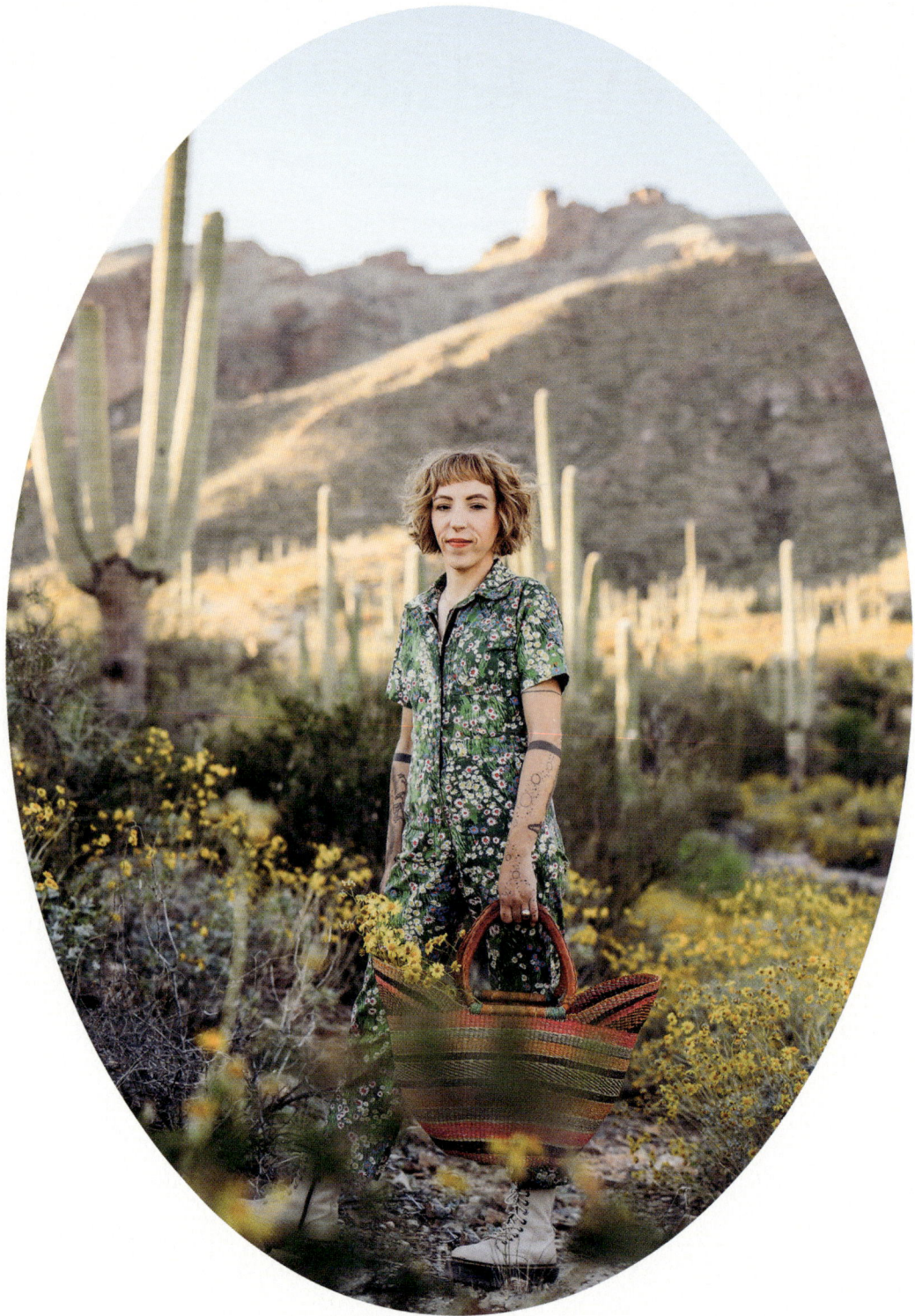

About the Author

Sonoran Rosie, also known as Rosie Crocker, lives in Tucson, Arizona, and grew up in the Sonoran Desert. She has worked with desert plants for ten years and started her desert botanical business, also called Sonoran Rosie, in 2017. Rosie loves to work to build community and spread awareness about the benefits of desert plants. She believes in fostering connection between people, the earth, and the desert to give power and meaning to our lives. Sonoran Rosie was started when Rosie discovered a lack of natural desert aromatherapy options. Inspired by local herbs like creosote, Rosie studied with a local herbalist and created hair, self-care, and skincare products that capture desert essence.

By foraging desert plants, Sonoran Rosie harnesses nature's properties for wellness and aromatherapy, while using sustainably sourced, organic ingredients and minimizing plastic use. A portion of proceeds support organizations like the Tucson Wildlife Center and the Coalition for Sonoran Desert Protection.

In 2022, Rosie opened Arizona Poppy in downtown Tucson to showcase the local maker community, offering handmade jewelry, ceramics, vintage items, potted plants, and more from over seventy local artisans.

First published in 2025 by Wellfleet Press,
an imprint of The Quarto Group,
142 West 36th Street, 4th Floor,
New York, NY 10018, USA
(212) 779-4972
www.Quarto.com

EEA Representation, WTS Tax d.o.o.,
Žanova ulica 3, 4000 Kranj, Slovenia.
www.wts-tax.si

Wellfleet titles are also available at discount for retail, wholesale, promotional, and bulk purchase. For details, contact the Special Sales Manager by email at specialsales@quarto.com or by mail at The Quarto Group, Attn: Special Sales Manager, 100 Cummings Center Suite 265D, Beverly, MA 01915 USA.

10 9 8 7 6 5 4 3 2 1

ISBN: 978-1-57715-527-0

Digital edition published in 2025
eISBN: 978-0-7603-9636-0

Library of Congress Control Number: 2025933911

Group Publisher: Rage Kindelsperger
Creative Director: Laura Drew
Editorial Director: Erin Canning
Managing Editor: Cara Donaldson
Editors: Katie McGuire and Flannery Wiest
Cover and Interior Design: Laura Klynstra
Cover and Interior illustrations: Hannah Davies
Author Photo: Lea Ortiz, Elle O Studio

Printed in Huizhou, Guangdong, China TT072025

This book provides general information on various widely known and widely accepted foraging practices and herbal remedies. However, it should not be relied upon as recommending or promoting any specific practice, recipe, or method of treatment for a particular condition, and it is not intended as a substitute for medical advice or for direct diagnosis and treatment of a medical condition by a qualified physician. Readers who have questions about a particular condition, possible treatments for that condition, or possible reactions from the condition or its treatment should consult a physician or other qualified health care professional and use appropriate precautionary measures when engaging in any foraging activity or use or consumption of organic materials.